THE
Caregiver's
Companion

THE
Caregiver's
Companion

Words to Comfort and Inspire

BettyClare Moffatt

BERKLEY BOOKS, NEW YORK

THE CAREGIVER'S COMPANION

A Berkley Book / published by arrangement with
the author

PRINTING HISTORY
Berkley trade paperback edition / March 1997

The Putnam Berkley World Wide Web site address is
http://www.berkley.com/berkley

ISBN: 0-425-15617-6

BERKLEY®
Berkley Books are published by The Berkley Publishing Group,
200 Madison Avenue, New York, New York 10016.
BERKLEY and the "B" design
are trademarks belonging to Berkley Publishing Corporation.

PRINTED IN THE UNITED STATES OF AMERICA

10 9 8 7 6 5 4 3 2 1

For my beloved mother, Helen Edwina Thomas Cook, and my beloved son, Michael Roy Welsch, who have taught me everything I know about caregiving, in gratitude and love. You have changed my life by your presence.

Contents

Ending the Caregiving

After the Caregiving

Appendix A: Legal Forms

Appendix B: Resource Guide

Introduction

"One of my colleagues in the field of caregiving once said, 'There are only four kinds of people in this world:

- *Those who have been caregivers,*
- *Those who currently are caregivers,*
- *Those who will be caregivers,*
- *Those who will need caregivers.'*

That pretty much covers all of us!"

—ROSALYNN CARTER
From *Catalyst* magazine,
Spring 1995

I have been a caregiver for many years. I am still learning to be a caregiver, even as I write these words, as my mother's four-year battle with terminal illness continues. I have walked this path before, with a son who died of AIDS, with a mothers' caregiver group, with hospices and hospitals and advocacy and support groups, through seven years of writing, editing, lecturing, and publishing in the fields of death and dying and grief recovery. I have witnessed the extraordinary courage of caregivers, both personal and professional, and their dedication to the people that they serve and love.

I have gathered together in this book bits and pieces of

what I have learned from my experience as a caregiver and writing other books on caregiving, recovery, and forgiveness.

To help you on your journey as a caregiver, I have also interviewed both professional and personal caregivers and their loved ones in order to present many different aspects of caregiving.

Time after time I have seen women and men exhausted, numbed, depleted, and grieving, with no idea how to switch gears—both during and after caregiving—to focus on their own care. It is as if all their emotions, time, energy, effort, prayers, and willing hands have been focused for so long on the needs of the loved ones they are caring for, that they leave nothing for themselves. This is more than tunnel vision. It's tunnel emotion. For caregivers, it sometimes seems inconceivable that there will ever be a time when life can go on as normal and the duties of caregiving will be over. We refuse even to imagine such a day, since that time coming would mean that our loved one will be gone.

Our society is often indifferent to the needs of the caregiver. Doctors and nurses focus on the patient. Friends and remaining loved ones are uneasy or in denial at our grief. Ministers speak bland promises of life hereafter. But what about our own lives hereafter, both during and after the caregiving? How do we go on? Is there a road map? Our primary role has been focused on others and their consuming and urgent needs. What can we do for ourselves? And how do we do it? I have known people who have taken care of their elderly parents, their spouses, their dying children. Sometimes all three. I marvel at their dedication, courage, compassion, patience, tirelessness. I marvel at the lessons of love that they embody for the rest of us. I marvel at their courage and their dignity. But I have seen—and experienced first-hand—how difficult it is both to continue with your own life during caregiving and to rebuild a new life afterward. This book will help you to do just that.

This book is divided into four sections: "Beginning the Caregiving," "Continuing the Caregiving," "Ending the Caregiving," and "After the Caregiving." Legal forms to help both the patient and the caregiver make wise decisions are reproduced in appendix A. A comprehensive resource guide, in appendix B, lists organizations that assist in caregiver recovery and each state's agencies on aging and insurance. Thus, health professionals and therapists, as well as the actual caregivers for whom this book is intended, will find this to be a useful resource. Throughout the book, inspirational ideas from other caregivers and health professionals serve as reminders of the positive healing journey that the reader is now creating for him- or herself.

The Caregiver's Companion comes out of my own experiences and the experiences of many, many caregivers I have known. I hope that it will serve as a compassionate and consoling friend and way-shower to caregivers who are learning how to care for themselves as well as for their loved ones.

This is your story as well as mine. I honor your journey through caregiving. Blessings!

—BettyClare Moffatt, 1997

THE
Caregiver's
Companion

Beginning the Caregiving

It is only with the heart that one can see rightly. What is essential is invisible to the eye.

—ANTOINE DE SAINT EXUPÉRY

Calling from the Mind and Heart

Once, when my mother was in the hospital for major surgery after badly breaking her hip, I went home from my daily vigil at the hospital to rest and prepare for an evening engagement. This was at the end of the third year of my mother's sojourn through Parkinson's disease. A host of other medical problems were affecting her, including the Parkinson's dementia that comes when the brain stem begins to disintegrate, and which shares many symptoms with Alzheimer's disease.

I was supposed to participate in a national fund-raising event for the homeless that night, the Writers Share Our Strength readings. Everything had been set up at a local bookstore for a two-hour reading of selected passages from my books and a discussion period afterward. Similar events were being coordinated all over the country.

As I stood in my bedroom, dressing for the event, tears kept rolling down my cheeks. Attempts at applying makeup were futile. My heart hurt.

Suddenly I thought I heard my mother calling me. But I had just left her bedside, not three hours before. Surely she couldn't need me again. I had work to do. I ignored the insistent yammering of my heart as long as I could. Finally I gave up. I called the coordinator of the event. I told him the situation. I told him that I could not keep my commitment to the readings. He understood perfectly and urged me to return to the hospital.

I walked into the hospital room. I don't know what I expected—that she had died during the time I was away from her, that she had been rushed to the emergency room. Surely there had been another crisis. My adrenaline was pumping. I was breathless.

My mother was sitting up in a chair by the bedside. Her face lit up when she saw me. She was clear, lucid. She was the mother I remembered from so long ago. The toll of Parkinson's, dementia, and major surgery semed to be arrested for a few moments in time. I bent over to kiss her. She jabbed a finger into my chest, right on the breastbone. "Calling from the mind and heart," she whispered. "Me to you."

We spent a couple of hours together, reminiscing about the wonderful times we had spent together over the years. My mother smiled often, tremulously. Her voice was weak. Her hands trembled. But the love between us was like two candle flames meeting. Mind to mind. Heart to heart.

When I left the hospital room, it was after nine o'clock. I walked outside into the cold, crisp, clear air. I breathed deeply. I looked up into the night sky, at all the stars that trembled, winking on and off. "'Calling from the mind and heart,'" I whispered to myself as I got into the car. "That's what we do. And the mind and the heart answer Yes."

Caregiver Concerns

In my conversations with caregivers, certain themes emerged that seemed common to all of them, whether they were family, friends, or health professionals.

- We sometimes fear that we will "catch death" if we are around the dying process and the dying person.

- Doctors and nurses and professional caregivers are taught detachment, and that very detachment can be a barrier, an armored defense against feeling and caring and understanding.

- Caregivers often make jokes to cover their own fear and pain.

- Survivors are often brushed aside and ignored by health professionals who are themselves afraid of death.

- Nursing schools don't teach you how to handle death and dying or the concerns of either the patient or the family.

- A death is often called "a good death," or "a terrible death"—societal judgments that perpetuate themselves.

- Not mentioning death does not mean it isn't there or that it will go away.

- We are taught to worship youth and strong, beautiful bodies, and so we save bodies at all costs, hooking them up to every possible machine until the life has gone out of the soul and the personality, and only a shell remains.

- One death experience can trigger other unresolved feelings of loss, which the caregivers must also work through.

- Death is the last taboo. We can now talk openly about sexuality, but not about death.

- People who work with death and dying often feel as though they are in a "war zone," and other people are "civilians" who don't understand.

- Despite increased lifespans we are all going to have to face our own death and the deaths of those we love.

- We are neither ghoulish nor sick ourselves if we work with sick and dying people; neither are we noble saints like Mother Theresa. We are just reaching out to do our part.

- We don't have to know everything about death in order to bear it and make the transition bearable for others. Yet our efforts to understand can help us live more peacefully in the world of both the flesh and the spirit.

- We don't have to be martyrs to serve well. We must continue caring for ourselves in order to avoid not only burnout and callousness, but also exhaustion and sickness of our own.

- Caregiving is often overwhelming, and when we nurse a dying spouse, family member, patient, or friend, there is no "reward" in the form of restored health—the end result is death.

- We must continually recharge and nurture our own self because life does indeed go on even as death goes on.

- It is all right— in fact, it is necessary—to take a vacation, a sabbatical, a breather. The work is still there whenever we are ready to return to it.

- Comfort is sometimes the only thing we can give, and it is enough.

- We don't need to argue or justify to others what we do or don't do. Acceptance of our own feelings and our own limitations helps us to be more compassionate and courageous.

- We must love ourselves as we love others if we are to be equal to the task.

- Death is neither a failure nor a punishment, but rather the last great journey we will take.

- We will indeed learn more, experience more, feel more, *be* more as we travel through the valley of the shadow of death. And we will live more and love more as we are changed by this passage.

Please Listen!

BY DR. RAY HOUGHTON
From *Stepping Stones to Grief Recovery*

When I ask you to listen to me and you start giving advice, you have not done what I asked.

When I ask you to listen to me and you begin to tell me why I shouldn't feel that way, you are trampling on my feelings.

When I ask you to listen to me and you feel you have to do something to solve my problem, you have failed me, strange as that may seem.

Listen! All I ask is that you listen, not talk or do—just hear me.

Advice is cheap; twenty-five cents will get you both Dear Abby and Billy Graham in the same newspaper.

And I can do for myself. I am not helpless. Maybe discouraged and faltering, but not helpless.

When you do something for me that I can and need to do for myself, you contribute to my fear and inadequacy.

But when you accept as a simple fact that I do feel what I feel, no matter how irrational, then I can quit trying to convince you and can get on to the business of understanding what's behind my irrational feeling.

And when that's clear, the answers are obvious and I don't need advice. Irrational feelings make sense when we understand what's behind them.

So please listen and just hear me. And, if you want to talk, wait a minute for your turn, and I'll listen to you.

When Someone You Love Is Ill

I was at a support group for caregivers when a new facilitator joined our meeting. I have seen how helpful and how kind experienced group leaders can be for the grieving; I have also noticed that the very impersonality of some psychological professionals can be a subtle barrier, one that they themselves are often unaware of.

This young counselor sincerely wanted to help. She had read all the literature on caregiving. She had obviously served her internship. But she started off the meeting by talking instead of listening.

She began by talking about our "caretaking duties." We listened politely for a few moments, waiting for new insights to emerge that would help to lift the cloud of fatigue and emotional overload that most of us were experiencing. But she went on and on. It sounded more like a lecture than a helping hand.

Finally a woman who was caring for her elderly mother spoke up.

"Please," she said, "Don't tell us about caretaking. We are not caretakers. Being a caretaker implies that you are guarding a house, polishing antiques, tending a garden. Caretaking means you are taking care of things and objects, keeping them pristine and safe from breakage.

"But I am not a caretaker," she continued. "I am a *caregiver*. There's a lifetime of distinction between those two words. I care for my mother, yes, but I give to her. I give to her out of conscious choice. And she is still dying, inch by inch, before my eyes. I cannot keep her immaculate or polished, or unbroken, or safe from the ravages of time. I can only give. And give some more. So if you must talk *to* me or *at* me, instead of *with* me, tell me how I can continue being a caregiver. For I will never be a caretaker."

The group was silent, hushed. The young health professional turned red and started to say something, then caught herself. She struggled for composure.

"You're right," she said quietly. "Thank you for correcting me. I'd like to know what I can do to help. I haven't walked in your shoes. I don't know what you need. But I do know, now, that you are all caregivers."

Are you a caregiver or a caretaker? Are you one who listens? Or one who tells others how they should or must feel, what they should or must do? Whether you are a family member caught up in the journey of your loved one's illness, or a helping professional, it is wise to stop and ask yourself often, "Am I a caregiver or a caretaker?" You will know the answer. You will continue onward then with more empathy, more compassion. Because you care. Because you give.

What Can I Do to Help?

The next time people ask you what they can do to help you in your caregiving responsibilities, tell them. Tell them specifically.

- "You can come and sit with Mother next Tuesday so that I can get out for a few hours."
- "You can drive me and my father to the doctor next Thursday, because I can't get him in and out of the car by myself without injuring my back."
- "You can pick up these prescriptions from the pharmacy once a week and bring them to my house." Or,

"You can pick up the walker from home health care."
Or whatever else you need.

- "You can arrange for someone to clean my parents' house once a month as a Christmas gift to them and to me."
- "You can bring food, books, or catalogs that list special clothing and devices to make my tasks easier or him more comfortable. Better yet, you can send away for some items, checking with me on our needs, and surprise him with your thoughtfulness."
- "You can take my mother to Bible study, the beauty shop, the grocery store, or just out for a drive, thus relieving me for a while and giving her an opportunity to get out of the house."
- To a family member, "All I want for Christmas is a few days for myself, with or without a vacation destination. As a gift to me and to Mother, can you come and stay with her for a few days?" Or, "Would you be willing to check on her daily in her home?" Or, "Could you please visit her in the nursing home?" Or, "Can you be available for emergencies so that I can go off without worry?"
- "Can you arrange Meals on Wheels and come by to see that she eats properly?"
- "Can you arrange transportation so that he can get to adult day care, physical therapy, or the senior citizens center while I work?"

These are just a few of the things that others can do, at various stages of the loved one's illness, to help the primary caregiver and the one who is ill. There are, of course, professional health care resources that can assist you. Some of these are listed in appendix A. But it takes time and effort to search out local health resources that specifically meet your loved one's needs at every stage of illness.

Family members can and must be encouraged to share the responsibility. Perhaps someone else in the family circle can be responsible for medical forms and claims and payments. Perhaps someone else can handle the legal aspects of a loved one's illness, whether it be an updated will, a durable power of attorney for health care, a living will, a guardianship or conservatorship, the sale of property, income taxes, or any other time-consuming monetary or legal problem. All these issues must be addressed, whatever the family dynamics may be. One person cannot do it all. Nor should one.

Having gone through more than one long-term caregiving experience, I strongly urge each new caregiver I meet, "Share the responsibilities. Share the care. Ask for help. And continue asking until you get it."

When a Friend Is Ill

Thanks to Chelsea Psychotherapy Associates, NYC, for permission to reprint this excerpt from "When a Friend Has AIDS." The authors are Dixie Beckham, Diego Lopez, Luis Palacios-Jimenez, Vincent Patti and Michael Shernoff.

When someone you know becomes ill, especially with a serious illness like AIDS or cancer, you may feel helpless or inadequate. If this person is a good friend, you may say, "Just call if you need anything." Then out of fear or insecurity, you may dread the call if it comes. Here are some thoughts and suggestions to help you help someone who is ill.

Try not to avoid your friend. Be there; it instills hope. Be the friend, the loved one you've always been, especially now when it is most important.

Touch your friend. A simple squeeze of the hand or a hug can let him or her know that you care.

Call and ask if it is okay to come for a visit. Let your friend make the decision. If he or she does not feel up to visitors that day, you can always visit on another occasion. Now is a time when your friendship can help keep loneliness and fear at a distance.

Respond to your friend's emotions. Weep with your friend when he or she weeps. Laugh when your friend laughs. It's healthy to share these intimate experiences. They enrich you both.

Call and say you would like to bring a favorite dish. Ask what day and time would be best for you to come. Spend time sharing a meal.

Go for a walk or outing together but ask about and know your friend's limitations.

Offer to help answer any correspondence that may be giving some difficulty or that your friend is avoiding.

Call your friend and find out if anything is needed from the store. Ask for a shopping list and make a delivery to your friend's house.

Celebrate holidays and life with your friend by offering to decorate the home or hospital room. Bring flowers or other special treasures.

Include your friend in your holiday festivities. A holiday doesn't have to be marked on a calendar; you can make every day a holiday.

Check in with your friend's spouse, carepartner, roommate, or family member. They may need a break from time to time. Offer to care for your friend in order to give the loved ones some free time. Invite them out. Remember, they may need someone to talk with as well.

Your friend may be a parent. Ask about the children. Offer to bring them to visit.

Be creative. Bring books, periodicals, taped music, a poster for the wall, home-baked cookies or delicacies to share. All of these can bring warmth and joy.

It's okay to ask about the illness, but be sensitive to whether your friend wants to discuss it. You can find out by asking, "Would you like to talk about how you're feeling?" However, don't pressure.

Like everyone else, a person with a serious illness can have both good and bad days. On good days treat your friend as you would any other friend. On the bad days, however, treat your friend with extra care and compassion.

You don't always have to talk. It's okay to sit together silently reading, listening to music, watching television, holding hands. Much can be expressed without words.

Can you take your friend somewhere? Transportation may be needed to a treatment, to the store or bank, to the physician, or perhaps to a movie. How about just a ride to the beach or the park?

Tell your friend how good he or she looks, but only if it is realistic. If your friend's appearance has changed, don't ignore it. Be gentle; yet remember, never lie.

Encourage your friend to make decisions. Illness can cause a loss of control over many aspects of life. Don't deny your friend a chance to make decisions, no matter how simple or silly they may seem to you.

Tell your friend what you'd like to do to help. If your friend agrees to your request, do it. Keep any promises you make.

Be prepared for your friend to get angry with you for no obvious reason, although you feel that you've been there and done everything you could. Remember, anger and frustration are often taken out on the people most loved because it's safe and will be understood.

Gossip can be healthy. Keep your friend up to date on mutual friends and other common interests. Your friend may be tired of talking about symptoms, doctors, and treatments.

What's in the news? Discuss current events. Help keep your friend from feeling that the world is passing by.

Offer to do household chores, perhaps taking out the laundry, washing dishes, watering plants, feeding and walking pets. This may be appreciated more than you realize. However, don't do what your friend wants and can do for him- or herself. Ask before doing anything.

Send a card that simply says, "I care!"

If your friend is religious, ask if you can pray together. Spirituality can be very important at this time.

Don't lecture or direct your anger at your friend if he or she seems to be handling the illness in a way that you think is inappropriate. You may not understand what the feelings are and why certain choices are being made.

A loving family member can be a source of strength. Remember that by being a friend you are also a part of the family.

Do not confuse acceptance of the illness with defeat. This acceptance may free your friend and give your friend a sense of his or her own power.

Talk with your friend about the future: tomorrow, next week, next year. It's good to look toward the future without denying the reality of today.

Bring a positive attitude. It's catching.

Finally, take care of yourself! Recognize your own emotions and honor them. Share your grief, anger, feelings of helplessness, or whatever is coming up for you, with others or a support group. Getting the support you need during this crisis will help you to be a real friend for your friend.

Forgiveness and Caregiving

This story originally appeared in a slightly different format in Journey Toward Forgiveness: Finding Your Way Home *(N.Y.: MasterMedia, 1995).*

Nowhere is forgiveness more misunderstood than in caring for a person who is ill and dying. Nowhere is heroism, self-sacrifice, and the practice of unconditional love more misused. Somehow we expect, as do our loved ones who have need of us, that the road to caregiving will lead us to a deeper understanding of both life and death, a deeper expression of love and solicitude. It will. It does. It also leads us to exhaustion, resentment, sometimes bitterness, and the opening up within us of every unhealed emotion we have ever held. I know. Words like rage, shame, grief, guilt, and fear take on intense emotional resonance when you are in the midst of caregiving. I have been there more than once. Caregiving is both a purifying process and a deep part of our spiritual journey. And it is difficult. It can kill us along the way if we are not aware. Our own expectations of ourselves can never match the heroic and super-human powers we are expected to possess and exercise on behalf of others, even as we go through our own dark nights of the soul.

My own experiences with caregiving started with the illness of my father. I was nineteen, with two babies in diapers, a husband who was overseas, and two younger sisters in school while my mother worked at her first job. When my father became too ill to be cared for at home, he would go to the Veterans Administration hospital, only to come home again to the back bedroom, where he suffered from constant nightmares that reverberated through the tiny tract home in which we all lived. I was very close to my father, and we grew even closer during the course of his illness, but I was young, emotional, and overworked, and by the end of his life, I was conscious only of a vast relief coupled with a great emptiness.

This was only the first of many opportunities to teach me about life in the midst of death. I struggled greatly later on, when the man I had been married to for eighteen years suffered from alcoholism and mental illness. He died three years after our divorce, bitter and enraged to the end, without ever forgiving me for leaving him.

By that time, however, I was fully engaged in the work of caring for my beloved son Michael through his two-year journey through AIDS. His legacy of love, the luminosity and sweetness of this dear young man who taught all his family lasting lessons of unconditional love and forgiveness, changed my life. For years I strove to do the work I felt that he would have done had he lived. It was a valuable, intense time for me. And I regret nothing of those seven years except that, looking back now from a more balanced perspective, I would have been kinder to myself. I would have found time for joy and healing and balance, as well as for this intense journey of the spirit.

As I write these words, I am engaged in my mother's long struggle with a debilitating and terminal illness. I am more tired than I have ever been. She has been ill for four years and the end is not yet in sight. I ponder the lessons I am still learning about caregiving and forgiveness. This time, I am learning that my body is no longer required to serve as a trauma center for others. No longer required to serve as a shock absorber for the painful illnesses of others. No longer a repository for their anguished emotions. I can love and I can serve. I still do. But finally, slowly, painfully, bit by bit, I am coming to learn the lessons of caregiving:

that I am a human being, not a superhuman savior; that I am engaged in my own journey of emotional and spiritual understanding; and that, yes, my emotions *do* matter, even in the midst of my loved one's terrible, insatiable, anguished needs.

And I must forgive myself for not being able to meet those needs. I must forgive myself. Perhaps you, too, are involved in a loved one's journey toward death. Perhaps you love this person with all your heart. And yet you may very well find that you are not able to do all and be all that you had hoped for when you began this exhausting and perilous journey. There are times when you can go no further. And there are times when you too must grieve. Grieve in the midst of the caring and the caregiving. At the beginning of my mother's battle with illness, I wrote a personal essay about my feelings. I was only beginning to come to terms with the knowledge not only that my mother was changing from the strong, cheerful, busy, independent woman she had always been, and that our roles were reversed (a common phenomenon when offspring care for their parents), but that I had lost my mother. Below is that essay.

Folding Sheets

My mother calls me on the phone, complaining. She wants me to come over and help her fold her sheets. The laundry has tired her. I go, of course. We fold the sheets together, to her command, inserting corners just so, stacking and pressing the creases.

When I see my mother these days, and I see her almost every day, I am struck with a wave of emotions—pity, terror, exasperation, and tenderness, coupled with a yearning, unfathomable love. She is a small bird now, in protective custody, where once she was a chirping, enthusiastic, busy, bustling sparrow.

"I miss my mother," she says to me as we fold the sheets. "I call out to her at night, and almost think I can see her form, vanishing down the hall. I miss my mother," she says again, and starts to cry.

My grandmother died on her seventy-ninth birthday, in her rocker, with the sun shining across her smiling face. My mother discovered her, just like this, when she came home from work. I remember that day.

Ten years ago, my mother held me as I cried into her arms that I was leaving my husband. Nine years ago my grandson died. We came to Mother's house from all across the country to lay him to rest. Eight years ago, my mother sent me off across the country to a new life, without recriminations. Seven years ago, my mother held me as my son lay dying. Six years ago, my mother came across the country to take care of her great-grandchildren. Five years ago, my mother sorted her memories of thirty years as I helped her leave her house, next-door to the house where her own mother had died, to move to a condo. Four years ago, my mother made the trek again to California, where she helped me move into new offices and living quarters. Three years ago, my mother staged a weekend family reunion and seventy-fifth birthday party for herself out in the countryside. She worked for weeks on this party. Sixty family members came to help her celebrate. Two years ago, my mother helped me move back from California and into a house near her. I was starting over. Again. I needed her. Now it is one year later. Now my mother has been diagnosed with a lingering, chronic, debilitating disease.

My mother cries for her mother. She is very close to the age when her own mother died.

What will I do? Oh I know what I will do *now*. I will fold sheets and get up on step stools to hunt for casseroles, and take her to the doctor, and clean her house, and bring food, and take her for outings. I will undo the zipper in the back of her church dress that she cannot reach, and kneel in front of her to guide her shoes onto her tiny feet. I will listen to her, and slow my steps to her faltering ones, and watch her as she dozes. But what will I do *then*?

My sons are scattered all over the country. They have busy lives. They will not come to help me fold my own sheets. Who will mother me? Who will help me when I cry out again, and again, and yet again, at the loss of the one person left in the world who loves me just as I am, without conditions, yet with great, unreachable expectations, and for all time and eternity? Who will love me forever, just as her own mother loved her? Who will comfort me?

I miss my mother.

As I write this book, I have no way of knowing whether my mother will still be alive for me to read it to her. Her mental faculties are going, even as her body stiffens and wastes away. She has become a frightened and confused child, so tiny, so weak, so needy, that it takes all my courage and all my love to be with her daily. And yet the love is there. "I will love you forever, Mama," I whisper to her as I kiss her good-bye.

Then I get into my car and drive away from the nursing home, and I ask for forgiveness. Why do I ask for forgiveness? Am I not doing all that a daughter can do? All that anyone can do? I ask for forgiveness because the human being that I am wants release for her and for me. I ask for forgiveness because I question the wisdom of her continu-

ing to live in so damaged a body and mind. I ask for forgiveness because I do not know God's will for all of us (my
sisters, my mother, and myself) in this terrible and exhausting time, and I struggle to understand these final and
irrevocable lessons of holding on and letting go, of loving
dearly and releasing the outcome.

Sometimes forgiveness is named by other words and attitudes than those customary. Sometimes it is called love.
Sometimes, it seems to me, it is called endurance. Sometimes it is called surrender.

I once interviewed Marianne Williamson, the well-
known spiritual teacher of A Course in Miracles, for an
earlier book I wrote on death and dying, called *Gifts for
the Living*. In the interview, she told me what to do when
someone is ill or dying:

> When you feel like "What can I do?" just know that your
> showing up and holding love in your mind means you are
> bringing the power of God. You are affecting the forces of
> comfort on an invisible level. God will do his part if you'll
> do yours. If you will just show up, he will tell you what to
> say, what to do, perhaps just sit there. You will be trans-
> formed through an attitude of service. Just don't run away.
> The only enemy is your tendency to want to shut down and
> run away. The only thing to fear is the fear itself. Just stand
> forth and ask God continually: "Open my heart and we'll do
> everything right."

I remembered Marianne's words, originally spoken to
me as we both worked within the AIDS crisis, when my
mother first became ill. I remember her words now, years
later, as I aim my car along its daily route, a route I could
now take with my eyes closed if need be, because it is so
familiar to me. The drive to my mother's last and smallest

place. I wonder each day if she will be lucid and loving, or lost in the terrible hallucinations that bewilder and terrify her.

"Just show up." The words echo in my mind. Just be there for her. Be the witness. Be the helping hand. Be the loving heart. Just show up.

I show up. Daily I show up. I hold my mother's hand. I struggle to understand the lessons of her life and the love she has taught me. I struggle to forgive. And I still miss my mother.

Forgiving the System

I asked a dear friend of mine, who has written books in the caregiving field and gone through her own long and terrible caregiving ordeal with her parents, to tell me of her experiences as a caregiver. Her father died of a stroke while taking care of her mother, who had Alzheimer's disease for many years before finally and mercifully dying about two years ago. My friend learned firsthand what it is to care for someone whose mental faculties are gone, but whose body needs care over a period of several years. I asked her to write out her thoughts on the subject of forgiveness. When she began, she found that now, long after the fact, her anger had centered on the system that thwarted her every attempt to get help for her parents, even while she had to continue to work as a full-time writer in order to support herself and to help them.

The most animosity I ever felt was against an institution, rather than a person. So that's what I will write about to answer your questions about forgiveness.

Dealing with local governmental bureaucracy was one of the most frustrating experiences I've ever had. My parents had been declared incompetent to look after themselves or to make their own decisions.

This particular staff was cold, authoritarian, unhelpful, and rigid, and in more than one instance, I was lied to. The case worker in charge told me that when I called in with information, I was to ask for her by number, not by her name. Can you believe that! I had to fight for months to get help for my parents. My father died of a stroke during this interminable process.

As I continued as the advocate for my remaining parent's long-term care needs, my anger coalesced against the system. As I mulled over all that had happened—and not happened—the situation itself became first the focus, then the turning point for my anger. I developed empathy for human beings whose work is so demanding and demeaning that they must be turned into automatons with numbers instead of names. I learned that bumping into situations and people who cause anger is unavoidable. It's just a part of life, even though it seems much more horrible when you are tired and full of frustration and sorrow yourself.

One of the ways we can deal with it is to take control of ourselves and our thinking and our emotions. The other is to play the cowboy bit and just punch them in the nose, which is a quick way to reach forgiveness because then the situation is quickly ended. My advice is to get the issue resolved as quickly as possible, then move on.

Finally I learned that I can only forgive myself for harboring any type of animosity against anyone, including the system. You remember when I threw the rocks in the ravine in order to release my resentments—you wrote

about it in "Throwing Stones" in your book *Soulwork*.*
[See section 4, "Ending the Caregiving."] Well, I know this
process helped you and a lot of other people. It helped me
too. When I threw the rocks, it was more of a release from
my own shortcomings at not understanding where the
other person was coming from. That's what I thought
about for a long time before releasing the rocks. In effect,
I forgave myself.

We all know that harboring anger is detrimental to one's
physical, emotional, and mental health. So get the anger
issue resolved as quickly as possible, that's my advice. And
don't forget to throw the stones. Hope this will help someone else who is going through what I went through.

Forgiveness works!

Preventive Forgiveness

*Another friend, who, like so many of my contemporaries,
had been involved for years with family needs and family
caregiving, gave me an intriguing insight on forgiveness.*

I think that one of the things that's most important to do,
when faced with caregiving, especially long-term, especially
with someone you love so much and who depends on you, is
to practice what I call preventive forgiveness. That's when
you have a good talk with yourself, or sometimes several
solitary conversations along the way, in which you remind
yourself that no matter how much you love the person you
are caring for, and no matter how much that person loves
you, there is no way you can meet all their needs. You can-

---

*See *Soulwork* by BettyClare Moffatt; Wildcat Canyon Press, 1994.
Co-published by New World Library.

not heal them, you cannot save them, you cannot make them happy, you cannot carry the pain and the fear for them. You are not responsible for their final journey and how they take it. Oh, that's a hard lesson to learn!

What I suggest for your own health and sanity (we all know stories of caregivers who have keeled over and died before the ones they were caring for), for your own peace of mind, is that you practice preventive forgiveness. That's when you forgive yourself now, today, every day for a while if need be, for not being able to meet all the needs of the person you love. There's a lot of talk these days about setting boundaries. Well, good luck to you if you can do that in a long-term caregiving situation. I have very seldom found that the caregivers don't give enough. But you know what? It's never enough. It can't be. The needs are too great. So you have to forgive yourself ahead of time so that you *can* go on, so that you *can* help. Get over your guilt fast. It's false guilt.

The truth is, no matter what you do, there's still going to be grief. There's still going to be remorse. There are still going to be the memories. The fatigue fades. The 'if onlys' will tear you apart if you let them.

Preventive forgiveness. Living and loving with an open, compassionate heart. Knowing you did the best you could, and it was enough.

Emotions and Caregiving

Somehow we think it's not all right to feel bad. The next book I write is going to be called I'm Not O.K. and You're Not O.K., and That's O.K.

Elisabeth Kübler-Ross,
M.D.

Over the years, I have collected stories of other caregivers, stories that help me to both understand and be kind to myself as I go through yet another caregiver journey. Some of these stories are harrowing and exhausting. Yet they are also filled with courage, compassion, and a fierce dedication to the loved one's journey. You are just beginning your caregiver journey. You will live your own story. You will meet your own lessons. But I would be remiss if I did not alert you, along this perilous yet rewarding path, of the emotions you will encounter along the way.

Please be kind to yourself as you wrestle with them.

ANGER

Most caregivers I know are not saints. They are human beings faced with an ongoing crisis. While no one doubts their love, they may in fact begin to doubt themselves as they face the anger that can simmer or erupt as they try their best to take care of a loved one's needs.

Sometimes we are angry at ourselves, for failing to be all that we think we should be, could be, and must be during this caregiving stint. Often we are angry at others, especially other family members, who will not or cannot share our load. Sometimes doctors, nurses, or "the system" are the culprits. There is plenty of blame to go around, especially when both financial and time needs cannot be met.

Often we are angry at God, for this great crisis thrust into our ordinary lives, an exhausting crisis that asks too much of us for too long, and for not answering our prayers for our loved one's recovery.

Later in this book, discussing the end of caregiving, I will address this painful issue of dealing with our feelings of God's abandonment. I seldom see this mentioned in caregiver literature.

Whatever our feelings at the beginning of our caregiver journey, rest assured that they will intensify. No matter how wise and mature we are, no matter how loving, no matter how resilient, we will be tested, often beyond our capacity, with the so-called negative emotions we may have spent a lifetime ignoring or suppressing.

"Anger can be a powerful tool for change," I wrote in *When Someone You Love Has AIDS,* about my son's death. "Anger can be a force that gets us up in the morning, that fuels us forward." You can use your anger to keep you going and to be the advocate for your loved one's care. You can learn to harness your anger so that it works for you, instead of suppressing it so much that it turns inward into depression, or taking it out on your loved one. And when the anger gets to be too much to handle (and it will), you can remove yourself from the situation temporarily (easier said than done, but it's better than exploding at the patient) and work through your anger privately, whether by screaming in the shower, talking a walk, or talking to a trusted friend or counselor—whatever it takes. Then the anger will not be so overwhelming. You may have to do this daily, and for a very long time.

GRIEF

Sometimes the anger turns into tears. That river of tears, which you sometimes may feel will never, ever stop, is an integral part of your coping.

With a long-term illness, there are layers of grief. There is anticipatory grief, in which you watch your loved one diminish and disintegrate before your eyes, and you not only mourn the person he once was, you mourn his illness step by step. You will eventually come to a place where either one or both of you—though seldom at the same time or on the same rhythm—can let go and move into acceptance. You become able to accept a merciful and kind death, with no more suffering, no more exhortations to keep on trying, keep on going, no more brave fronts that conceal the intensity of your despair, no more cheerful smiles that deny the reality of dying. You will grieve along with your loved one, remembering the good times, stringing memories like a garland of blessings. You watch him move away from a heroic struggle into an even more heroic peace. And when your loved one dies, as indeed he must, you will grieve alone. Until your grief is transformed in the next stage of your life, just as death transformed him.

FEAR

My experience has been that fear occurs mostly at the beginning of the caregiver journey. You fear that you will not be strong enough, or loving enough, or brave enough to do what needs to be done to help your loved one. Perhaps there is also, for many of us, a fear of illness, a fear of dying.

My mother, who had been so helpful and had coped so well with the deaths of her mother, her father, her brother, her two sisters, her husband, her grandson, and her great-grandson, became terrified of death and dying when she was incapacitated with Parkinson's disease. As the years passed and her condition worsened, she lived in increasing terror. No family member, minister, or counselor could alleviate her fear; it was unreasoning and controlling. It robbed her of years of peace and acceptance and love.

Elisabeth Kübler-Ross, the well-known pioneer in death and dying studies, postulates five stages that a person who is terminally ill must go through. These are denial, anger, bargaining, depression, and acceptance. You too will go through these five stages. You too will feel the emotions that your loved one feels. You too will work through layers of denial, anger, bargaining, depression, and acceptance. These stages do not occur in a strict order. They overlap and double back and keep on coming around again and again as the ill person and the people around her work through their feelings about illness and death.

But some people never do work through their emotions. They stay stuck in an agony that to me seems far worse than the actual death itself. Because you love the one you are caring for, and want so much to alleviate her pain, you may want your loved one to hurry up and work through her emotions and get to a more peaceful place. But just as the ill person cannot control her illness or her eventual death, so too you cannot. You must try not to control her emotions, her way of working through her fear. Expectations, unreasonable or otherwise, serve no useful purpose. Far better for you to heal your own fears than to try to influence someone who is going through the most intense and private period of her life, to do it the way you want.

Some people do not die a good death. Some people's personalities change so drastically when faced with a long-term, debilitating illness that those around them are shocked and bewildered. Your task is to comfort and to love and to accept your loved one's needs and expressions of those needs as much as you are able to at different stages of this journey. This is a heroic task indeed. It will teach you far more about human nature than you ever envisioned. It will help you work through your own fears to reach your own acceptance.

Caregiving is a shared journey. You are both in this stream of time and emotion, holding each other's hand. Sometimes you will just have to take a deep breath, walk away for a short while, and come back with your own feelings, including your fears, harnessed to an energy that serves. You will learn to "fear forward" into the next step of your caregiver journey. You will need to honor your emotions, whatever they may be at any given moment. Impatience will come, as will frustration, anxiety, disappointment, and sometimes an intense and overwhelming need to control the situation. But this is not a situation that can be controlled, and you must learn this hard lesson too. Again and again you will learn it.

GUILT

Guilt serves no purpose. Guilt is useless, demoralizing, exhausting beyond belief. Yet we all feel it. I hope you will face your guilt with as much courage as you face your fears. I hope that you can learn to let reason walk along with unreasoning guilt. Or else guilt will destroy you. For you will never, ever be able to meet all of your loved one's needs. You will always remember times in the past when you could have done it differently, or better, or with more kindness.

But now you have a new opportunity. Not to be the perfect daughter or son, parent, spouse, or caregiver. Now you have the opportunity to heal the wounds of the past, the things you have done that you ought not to have done, no matter how trivial or how tragic, or the things you have left undone. Now you have a chance to hold your loved one and let him or her know that all is well between you.

Sometimes this is a one-sided journey. Sometimes only you will heal. As the caregiving journey progresses, you will meet others, in this book and on the journey itself, who have their own stories to tell of guilt, that most insidious and demoralizing of emotions, and how they overcame it.

I will never forget the many times that my mother, who knew no other way, tried to manipulate her daughters through guilt. It didn't work. We were all doing what we could for our mother, according to what we felt best in the situation. It was hard sometimes not to judge either our mother or each other, but we learned not to let a guilt trip keep us from our primary goal, that of helping and loving our mother.

Just as there are predictable stages of the caregiver journey, so too are there stages of anger, grief, fear, and guilt. As you read the stories of other caregivers and how they coped, I hope that you will find insights and reassurances that will help you to continue.

Continuing the Caregiving

Through the resource of power we are able to show up. Through the resource of love we are able to pay attention to what has heart and meaning. Through the resource of vision we are able to give voice to what we see. Through the resource of wisdom we are able to be open to all possibilities and unattached to outcome.

—ANGLES ARRIEN

From *A Grateful Heart*

Managing the Caregiving

Once the initial shock of your loved one's diagnosis has passed, once you and your loved one and family and friends have gone through the first stage of dealing with the illness, the most practical thing you can do for your loved one is to help him or her make a plan for the journey. There will probably be lots of resistance on both sides, for who wants to face what may come later? But if terminally ill people's wishes are to be respected, it is wise for them to have as much decision-making power and choice as they can for as long as they can. Almost everyone wants to stay in their own home and be surrounded by the familiar outlines of their life. But along the way, hard decisions must be made.

Someone has to be the project manager. It is an integral part of the primary caregiver's task. At first, care may be piecemeal, but soon more care may be needed than any one person can provide. That's when it is time to call in every family member and encourage them, no matter how busy or reluctant or scared they may be, to share in the care of the loved one. This is easier said than done. You will always find that one person does more, and that as a long-term illness progresses, formerly supportive friends and relatives tend to fall by the wayside, while you, dizzy with fatigue, continue. But ask for help and continue to ask for help. No one can be the sole source of support for an ill person, no matter how much you care. Stories of caregivers who collapse and are hospitalized or die while their loved one continues to live are common in the annals of caregiving literature. You're in for a long haul. Conserve your strength.

One caregiver friend of mine, who is an eminently practical woman, offered me some advice. "Enlist the doctor, the nurses, the care attendants, the home health care people, the therapists, all as a team. Establish a good relationship with the primary physician and all who work for him. Together you can manage your mother's care more easily than if you try to go it alone, only calling on the doctor in the middle of an emergency."

Often it is the doctor or his nurse who will smooth the red tape with insurance and Medicare, and alert you to facilities and alternate care options. The Home Health Care people we worked with were wonderful. They assigned a social worker to take charge of my mother's case, to visit and explain to both my mother and her nearby family members how the system worked, and help my mother to make the decision to first go with Home Health Care, Meals on Wheels, and Occupational Therapy in her home, and then, when she could no longer live in her home, helped her to make the decision to move into an assisted-care facility.

Your case may be different. None of it is easy. But at each step of the journey, we called upon every health care professional we knew, and we enlisted emotional support for my mother through her church and her church friends. Each time my mother's declining health necessitated another move (a tremendous hardship on her physically as well as emotionally, but we had no choice), I made it a point to get to know each aide and nurse and helper on the various shifts of the various facilities. I would introduce myself each day, get to know their names, ask how my mother had done, ask how the family could best help. I would thank the attendants for their continuing labor and treat them with courtesy. It sounds like a small and rather obvious thing, but it is so important. I would tell them that

I would be there daily and wanted to work with them for the best outcome for my mother.

I noticed that when family members seldom visited a patient or took no time to get to know the staff, the care of the patient suffered. Sometimes it was only in small ways, but there was a difference, nevertheless. A friend of mine, who managed her mother's best friend's care in the hospital and a short-term rehab facility, saw firsthand how indifferent an ordinarily caring staff could be when there was no one around to ask the right questions and smooth away the difficulties of an elderly person adjusting to new circumstances.

My friend owned her own company and her work was demanding. Yet she coordinated her friend's care, a task that required meeting after meeting to straighten out all the little things that can happen when a large facility with three shifts of health care workers are involved.

Once a nurse spoke to my friend irritably when she asked about obtaining hot chocolate or at least hot water so that she could fix a night snack for her friend. Her friend weighed only eighty pounds and needed special snacks to keep up her strength.

"There are three hundred people in this facility, and we can't be going around giving special treatment to anyone," the nurse snapped back.

My friend persisted. "I will fix whatever she needs," she said. "I was only asking for information. You may have three hundred people to care for, but my mother's friend is the one I am caring for, and so I will continue to make her stay here as pleasant as possible."

My own experience with my mother's care has been different. After all the horror stories I had heard about nursing homes, and after being guided by the social worker and NurseFinders to find both the best assisted-living facility

and the best long-term care center, I was pleasantly surprised to find so many caring people involved. Granted,
there were always one or two whose personalities occa-
sionally clashed with the residents, but I never saw anyone
handled roughly or talked to in a condescending or pa-
tronizing fashion. Instead, I saw dedicated people, sometimes paid very little to do unpleasant and tiring work, who
seemed genuinely to care about the fate of the elderly assigned to their care. Some were more professional than
others, but they all tried to be cheerful and patient under
demanding circumstances. Sometimes I did not see how
they kept their patience.

But the system works both ways. Another friend of
mine, whose mother was in a long-term care facility, was
taken aback when she found her mother berating the aide
who cared for her needs. Her mother had always been a
courteous and pleasant woman, a well-bred Southern lady
who had instilled manners into my friend from her earliest
childhood. Yet my friend witnessed her mother calling the
aide her maid, ordering her around like a servant, and, on
another occasion, actually throwing her pills into the face
of the nurse who had come around to give her medication.

My friend was aghast. "You can't treat people that way,
Mother," she scolded. "They are here to help you. The very
least you can do is be pleasant." One new nurse-in-training
was crying as she left the room and my friend pointed this
out to her mother. "How do you expect people to help you
when you are rude and inconsiderate to them?"

"You apologize for me," said her mother. "You always
take their sides, anyway. You're all against me."

"No, Mother, it is you who must apologize," her daughter said firmly.

"But I'm the victim here," wailed her mother. "I'm the
one who's sick." What a telling statement!

"You're not a victim, Mother, and neither are these people who care for you. You're all in this together. You had better make friends with them. You need them more than they need you."

Later her mother apologized to the staff, in tears that she had hurt their feelings. Later still, one young woman who was responsible for bathing and dressing the patient said to the daughter, "I know your mother doesn't mean what she says. It's hard for her. I just remember my own grandmother and how it was with her. But thanks. Everyone likes to be treated right."

Whether your loved one is spending a short time in the hospital or a long time in a care facility or still receiving assistance at home, smooth the waters as best you can. You need all the help you can get, and everyone, as the young aide said, likes to be treated right.

On the other hand, if your loved one is not receiving the care she or he requires, don't hesitate to bring it to the attention of those in charge, or to move the patient to another facility. One of my friends had installed her mother-in-law in an expensive, prestigious facility. When she would visit at hours out-of-the-ordinary, she found that her mother-in-law was disoriented, sleeping an inordinate amount of time, and missing her meals. She believed that her mother-in-law was being overmedicated. She spoke to the people in charge, but the situation continued. My friend quickly moved her mother-in-law to another, smaller, less opulent facility, but one designed especially for the care of Alzheimer's patients. Her mother-in-law lived there for five years, until she died in her sleep. My friend said it was the best move she ever made.

So it is vitally important that at each health care step, all the people involved work as a team for the best good of the patient.

Surviving Triple Caregiving

I have a friend who has taught me a great deal about car-
ing for others. Whenever I feel that my own caregiving sit-
uation is hopeless and interminable, I call my friend. Her
practical advice sees me through. She is a way-shower. She
is also a formidable caregiver.

Connie is an only child, married to another only child. She
had taken care of family duties and responsibilities for her
mother and her mother-in-law, two widowed women, and
had a full-time career as a school guidance counselor. She
is a natural caregiver—practical, calm, solid, patient, tire-
less, and devoted. Her relationships with both her mother
and her mother-in-law were of loving acceptance mixed
with occasional exasperation. A loving marriage of almost
forty years and a grown son completed her life.

She retired early from the school system, planning to ac-
company her husband, a contractor, as his business took
him to small towns around Texas on three- and six-month
contracts, a necessity born of the recession. Connie
planned to paint (she had been a promising artist as a
young woman), explore the small towns with her husband,
and set up housekeeping at each stop, as if they were care-
free newlyweds again. One week after she retired, with a
deposit already in place on an apartment in a town some
two hundred miles away, her mother-in-law set fire to herself and her kitchen in the bewilderment and confusion of
Alzheimer's disease. Three days later, her mother broke
her hip.

Connie moved both mothers into her home, once their
short-term hospital stays were over. "There I was, fixing
three meals a day and watching TV with two old ladies,

who drove me crazy from morning to night. I'd just get one meal cleaned up, one bathroom cleaned up, one of them dressed, fed, and watered, when it would be time for medication or entertainment. I loved them both dearly, but they exhausted me with their demands. Eventually my mother-in-law was moved to an assisted-care community, then to a special Alzheimer's care nursing home. I vowed that my mother, one of the sweetest and dearest ladies in the world, would want for nothing. She lived in my home with me for five years, and made eighteen or twenty hospital visits for emergency procedures for her heart. In the midst of all of this, my husband was diagnosed with lung cancer and given less than six months to live.

"I cannot yet express to anyone the depth of my anger and despair. I remember regretting so bittterly that we had not had more time together during the last two years, when he had traveled on construction projects and I had been stuck at home caring for two invalids. That's when I vowed we would have one last vacation together. At the time, my mother-in-law was still living with my mother and me at our home. I hired a sitter, alerted friends as backup, and my husband and I took one last trip together. We went to a place in the mountains of New Mexico that had been our refuge and getaway for many years. He died a couple of months later, after putting all his business affairs in order. Thank God we had that time together! It sustained me through the long winter that followed.

"The day after my husband's funeral, I opened his construction company for business as usual. This surprised everyone in the business community, who thought that I would close his business and retire to take care of the remaining members of the family. But I didn't. I needed to make a living. At first I took my mother with me to work, learning the business while taking care of her. Later I hired a full-time housekeeper and companion for her. This released me to operate the business as the new president of the company. I had always had a good head for mediation, counseling, and helping other people. Now I found that I had a good head for business as well. My mother lived with me until she died at eighty-nine years of age. I never regretted taking care of her, but the last years took their toll. A year later, my mother-in-law died in her sleep at the nursing facility. I remember an enormous sense of relief, mixed with a feeling of joy that she would be reunited with her husband and son.

"When people ask me 'How did you do it?' I answer that I really don't know. Looking back, I probably would have done it a little bit differently. I would have hired sitters earlier and gone with my husband on his travels and had two more precious years together, instead of spending five years taking care of elderly relatives. I thought that I not only had to do it all, but that I could do it all. In large measure, I've succeeded.

"Now my friends come to me for advice and comfort as they face the same journey with their loved ones. I listen, and tell them that they will get through, not to twist themselves up with guilt over what they can and cannot do. I remember that after my mother-in-law and mother died I bought myself a new car and started taking a lot of weekend trips. I have family on both sides scattered all over the country. I kept on running the business, but I took more time for myself. I was one of the lucky ones. I had a supportive husband, I had retired from the school system, and there was enough money for everything from housekeepers to nursing homes. Most women I know are not so lucky. But when I look back, even I wonder how it was possible to do it all—and for five years. I'm glad it's over. I'm still here. I'm looking forward now to what I can do for me."

Stories from the Other Side
of Caregiving

FAMILY ANGELS AND GENTLE GHOSTS

My mother wrote this story shortly after she was diagnosed with Parkinson's disease, and was still living in her own home. She contributed it in a longer form to my book Opening to Miracles: True Stories of Blessing and Renewal. *Although she is a devout and traditional churchgoer, angels did not appear to my mother at the end of her life. Instead, what she called "gentle ghosts" came to help her through months of crisis. Whenever I read this story, I am struck by her own gentleness and faith. Later in her illness, my mother's personality changed completely, and in her mental and emotional confusion she no longer had access to her family angels, her gentle ghosts. Perhaps your loved one also has access, at some point in his or her illness, to the comfort of family angels and gentle ghosts. Perhaps this story will comfort both you and your loved one.*

This is reprinted from Opening to Miracles *with the generous permission of Wildcat Canyon Press.*

Having been a secretary for many years, I deal in business facts, not fantasy. I'm probably the most practical and down-to-earth person you'll ever meet. The only fantasy movie I ever went to was *E.T.,* and I cried my way all through that one, along with my grandchildren.

So I never expected, in fact, I was thoroughly surprised when a trio of gentle ghosts established themselves in my home.

I had been somewhat despondent for months, worrying

over all the things the doctor had told me, as I wasted away for no reason, or so the doctors said after each round of lab tests. But at least I had all my faculties, or so I told myself and my close friends. I tried to joke about my condition, as I ended more than one conversation with the wail of a child, 'I want my mother.' "

My friends laughed, but I often went home thinking about the closeness between my beloved mother and me in all the years in which she cared for me, and all the years I cared for her too. Even though we said good-bye at the cemetery, I thought of her every day and quoted all her little sayings she was so fond of telling me.

Well, she must have heard me. She must have heard the panic beneath my cry for help, because several weeks later, as I entered my apartment, I knew instantly that my mother was there. I couldn't catch her scent, for she never wore perfume. And I couldn't quite catch sight of her in any of the rooms of my apartment. But I knew she was there. Without a doubt, I knew that my mother was there. There was an aura of a fire in a fireplace just extinguished. That's the best way I can put it. A glow of love. I could feel my mother's love surrounding me, cherishing me. Although I could not quite catch a glimpse of her I just knew she was there, so close, so sweet, so near and dear.

I sat down in the first chair I touched. Then I sank down into the warmth of love surrounding me. I just let myself be in the light and love of her presence. Soon I was conscious of two other presences as well. I did not see any clothing or bodies. No one spoke.

Soon I gave up wondering about all of this and just allowed myself to feel the presence of my dear mother and the other two gentle ghosts.

How I wish that I could say that I could really see my

dear mother in the flesh or touch her or have her touch me. But that was not to be. Not yet, anyway.

This was not a life after death experience that you read about. There was no steady beam or brilliant light leading me onward through a dark tunnel, no hovering above the surgery table, no knowing for a moment or two that I had indeed died and seen God.

But my prayers were answered. I cried out for my mother and she came to me. This was a miracle to me. She came to me again and again. I even feel her presence now, as I write these words. This may not be your everyday miracle, but it has put me in the believers' corner for what is left of my life.

Soon I figured out that the other two gentle ghosts that had taken up residence in my home were my younger sister and my only brother.

I don't really know why God sent my brother and sister to my home to be ghosts as well. I wasn't particularly close to my brother as we grew up, but he didn't have long to be a young man anyway, as his Air Force plane crashed in World War II on a training flight just two days after his marriage. He was only eighteen years old. It was a long time ago. But I remember him always as a lean, smiling, mischievous boy with sparkling blue eyes, who teased me sometimes, yet never made me cry. He was always ready to help me do my hard chores. I'm afraid I even took advantage of his good humor. Once in a while in the evenings, as we sat on the big front porch in the house we all grew up in, I was aware of his presence close to me. He made me feel safe.

I'm seventy-seven years old now. My younger sister died about five years ago at the age of sixty-two. Lately she has been visiting me too, almost every night. Whenever I see her, she looks about eight years old. She's carrying her doll. I know it's her by the Buster Brown bobbed haircut we all wore back in those days, and by the pink ribbon in her hair. She spends most of her time crouched on the carpet in front of my TV set, slowly rocking her baby doll.

Whenever I go for a snack at bedtime, I call out to my brother and sister (I can see and hear them plain as day, even though I can only *feel* the presence of my dear mother at my side), "Anyone for ice cream, or cookies and milk?" They don't answer me, but they make a lot of noise on their own, just to let me know that they are here, keeping me company. But nobody rushes to the kitchen with me, so I believe I have learned one thing about my gentle ghosts, or you can even call them my family angels instead. It's just this. They have no real bodies, at least not on visits to earth.

I wonder if God lets angels come to earth at their favorite age, or at the age to do the most good in the assignment they have been given? I wonder. Sometimes I awaken to hear my mother's laughter, as well as the noises of my other two gentle ghosts. I will turn to say something to her, only to find that she has disappeared. I also used to look for my older sister to talk to, as she was the most fun of any of my family. But so far she hasn't shown up. Maybe she is busy elsewhere.

I am comforted to think that if God sent my mother to me because I cried out for her, then she was evidently supposed to give me encouraging thoughts about this sickness of mine. So I thank you, God, for my mother. And for the presences of my sister and brother too. I feel like they have moved in for the duration. Sometimes I feel selfish if I eat in front of them. Once, as I walked out of the kitchen with the cereal I had fixed for breakfast, I said loudly, "Help yourself." But there was no answer. Yet I know they are loving and protecting me. Sometimes they go away for a day or two, but then they come back.

Now I understand the phrase in 1 Corinthians, 'that now we see through a glass darkly, but soon we shall see face to face.' So I have been blessed. The promise is there. Soon I will see them face to face. I will see them and we will embrace one another. So I am comforted by my gentle ghosts.

It is just as easy to believe in gentle ghosts as in fierce, terrifying hauntings. And if the gentle family ghosts of the past can come into our present awareness, they can help you and me to prepare for the future as they helped my mother. They can both comfort and console us. If there is indeed no time and no space for angels to conform to, then my friend's gentle family angels can and will continue to surround her with their loving presence, and guide her safely home into her dear mother's arms.

ALL OF THE LAUGHTER, ALL OF THE TEARS

Deborah Roth is a well-known writer, editor, ordained Interfaith minister and grief counselor. She has served on the staff at the Center for Help in Time of Loss as communications director and facilitator of the Healing through Humor support group. She is the author of Stepping Stones to Grief Recovery *and* Being Human in the Face of Death, *where this story originated in slightly different form.*

There is nothing like facing your own death to show just how human you really are. Before it happened to me, I thought I had a fair handle on dying. After all, I'd worked at the Center for more than five years, and I had certainly tried to look inside and confront my fears about death and loss. But when the report came back indicating that I had breast cancer, nothing was like I thought it would be. I was on the examining table when the doctor told me and I just stared at him. This wasn't supposed to be happening to me.

"Are you all right?" he asked.

"I guess it's back to the drawing board," I said, realizing my concept of "how it was" was no longer valid. I couldn't sort out the many feelings that were going on, but I knew that one of the strongest was a sense of failure, as if somehow I'd flunked life or done something wrong.

I think being a part of the Center for Help in Time of Loss, surrounded by caregivers, gave me a special problem. I had a strong reluctance to assume the role of "helpee." I wanted to share my feelings, but I was furious at the slightest hint that I needed help because it made me feel like a lesser person, somehow weak and vulnerable. Any phrase like "I hear you" that smacked of the therapeutic method made me absolutely crazy. These were my friends and they were also professionals and the two didn't seem to gel.

I became aware of the real value of having someone outside family and friends as a line of support. I felt the rise of that invisible barrier between the well and the sick, and I was outraged by it. As you may have already guessed, I was not easy to be around. I think it's fair to say that prior to this experience, I was not given to temper tantrums and was considered, if perhaps a bit stubborn, pretty easy to get along with. What the diagnosis of cancer did was remove the lid on my emotions. It was like being on a roller coaster and everything seemed exaggerated: normal impatience became childish rage, spontaneity and playfulness took on a tinge of hysteria. Fear can do that. I think my intensity scared everyone, including myself. I'm not sure that being in caregiving always makes us worse patients, but I suspect there is some correlation. Maybe it's that health care "managers" are particularly insulted to discover what way down deep they always knew: human beings are in control of very few things, and life and death are mysteries that cannot be handled by formulas and rules.

From my all too human perspective clouded by fear, I was given a new view of the world of health care and it appeared as distorted as Alice's Wonderland. I was sitting in a radiology room of a large New York teaching hospital. I was being photographed so the radiologist could find the correct area to inject a blue dye that would mark the site of the biopsy for the surgeon. A routine mammography had picked up some suspicious cells and since there was no palpable tumor, the location had to be pinpointed by another method. The young woman who was attempting to get the right picture was pleasant, but harried. Above the machinery I spotted a poster on the wall that shouted:

BREAST CANCER, THE DREADED DISEASE!

"Who put that up?" I asked.

"Oh, the hospital administration, I think," she said.

"That's pretty stupid," I told her.

"Yeah, but they want it there," she said.

At that exact moment the door opened and a middle-aged doctor entered, accompanied by a young assistant. The older one had an accent that turned out to be Hungarian, but to me it immediately called up Auschwitz. I caught the last few words he was speaking to his student. "Ya, wasn't he a nice, benign man," he was saying.

"Benign, benign," I called out. "Keep that thought in mind." The two doctors looked at me curiously, as if to say, "Did I hear a voice coming out of that body?"

Not allowing themselves to be distracted, the younger one asked, "How much dye will you inject?"

Before his teacher could reply, I piped up. "Yoo-hoo, do

you see me? There's a person in here," I said, pointing to the middle of my chest.

Only the younger one looked up. "Oh, this is just technical stuff," he said. "You wouldn't be interested."

The procedure was painless, and the doctors were so pleased to have hit the right spot on the first try that I just retreated inside myself, until the younger man said, "You can go to Admitting now."

"I don't know where it is," I said. My voice quivered and suddenly he seemed to notice me.

"Is something the matter?" he asked.

"I'm scared," I said.

"Oh," he said. "I don't know where it is either, but I'll go with you."

I felt a lump of tears in my throat at the first sign of recognition.

We found our way up a back staircase, and he turned me over to an admitting nurse.

"You're late!" she barked. My young doctor friend looked as confused as I did. I could hear the White Rabbit, "You're late, you're late, for a very important date. . . ."

Two weeks later, I was back in the same hospital coming out of anesthesia after a mastectomy. Somebody had his head very close to mine and his face was tight-lipped with rage. "I don't enjoy being called kid," he said. I must have insulted him while I was under.

"I'm sorry," I said, "I don't know what happened, but the anesthesia must be making me feel paranoid," I offered.

"You don't just *feel* paranoid," he said. "You *are* paranoid."

The next thing I heard was a woman's voice, softly reprimanding me.

"You're not behaving nicely at all," she said. "You're snapping at everyone."

I have no idea what I had been saying or doing, but as I came awake I was wary, and I made a firm decision after that to say as little as possible. Over the next few days in the hospital, as I waited to learn if the cancer had spread to the nodes and if I would need chemotherapy or any further treatment, I came to a conclusion about whether or not I wanted to buck what seemed to me an indifferent and insensitive system. This is not to say that many nurses weren't kind, and in fact my own surgeon was particularly understanding and compassionate—characteristics not often attributed to his profession.

One thing he told me was extremely calming. I had been wondering, as is often the case, what I had done physically or emotionally that might have caused the disease. The surgeon was just leaving my room when he turned back to face me. "If you learn one thing from me and one thing only," he said, "you didn't do anything wrong. So many patients feel guilty and guilt is a waste of time."

Of course it's natural to want to find a cause so that you can feel there is a way to prevent a reoccurrence. Taking responsibility for your health can be useful, and anything that takes away the "victim mentality" seems to me to be helpful. But—and it's an important "but"—guilt for the past can be just as harmful and imprisoning. All of this is to say that I saw much that was humane and caring in the medical field, but the pressure and bureaucracy in the hospital created an often inhuman atmosphere. My conclusion, however, was to accept what I was not about to change. There was no way I could see to make a dent in the hospital system and my own choice would be to get out of there as soon as possible. It crossed my mind that maybe the hospital experience shouldn't be all that wonderful—what if it was such an appealing place that nobody wanted to leave? No, I'd settle for escape and leave the reform to others.

The pathology report was like a pardon from the governor. The nodes were all negative and there was no evidence of cancer anywhere—it had all come out in the mastectomy. There would be no chemotherapy. Although I would be considered high risk from now on, and under scrutiny, I experienced a wild sense of freedom. In fact, wildness seemed to dominate the months before and after the mastectomy.

If I was a little taken aback by my own behavior, I saw how it really troubled my family and friends. The child in me had emerged and would not be denied. The line between childlike and childish was blurred. I remember one of my closest friends becoming teary just before I went into the hospital.

"I just realized that I might lose you," she told me. "I could imagine you saying, 'Take that trip we planned together—do it for both of us.'"

My reaction was to go berserk. "Forget that scene," I shouted. "If I'm going to die, why don't you come with me!"

Another friend who had been endlessly patient with me finally threw up her hands when I refused to rest on my first day home, going directly to a class at the seminary where I was studying to become an Interfaith minister. I couldn't wait to show my fellow students and the teacher that I was alive and well. I remember one man coming up to my table at lunch after class and whispering in my ear, "You're a true warrior."

That was what was so puzzling. I think I was both courageous and outrageous—a warrior and a brat.

I even speculated briefly on whether this whole experience wasn't some unconscious way for me to express my courage. It was certainly the first time I ever felt validated as a person who stood up under fire. All my other life battles, like divorce, loneliness, and aging, were private ones that were rarely seen or acknowledged.

On the other hand, my impatience and my outbursts were startling. I was sure that such behavior was uncharacteristic and disappointing to those who felt they knew me better. "She's not herself," was, I think, the general conclusion. For sure I wasn't acting the way I usually did.

My six-week recovery period was mostly wonderful. And at least a few things fell into place. For the first time that I can remember, I followed only my inner direction, which was actually the advice of my doctor. "Rest when you are tired, eat when you are hungry. You're your own best guide." I seemed to need very little sleep, but when I was tired I went right off without a thought.

I was also obsessed with rearranging furniture and adding plants and light to my room. I even went in search of an indoor fountain so that I could have the sense of being near water in a city apartment. Each new thing I added to the decor seemed to require a shift in the balance. A new ashtray made a lamp look out of place, a new pillow changed the color flow. What seemed like a simple diversion into decorating gave me a new perspective on this human experience.

I felt in the deepest core of myself an urge toward integrity. I felt there was a rightness to all things, based on balance and wholeness. It seemed as if each of us had a canvas to work on representing our lives, on which we could attempt to keep that balance intact. I was aware that I had worked hard to form a self-image that would be pleasing to others and myself. Make nice, don't be selfish. If uncomfortable feelings intrude on the picture, cover them over. Maybe rework a piece over here and then balance it over there, but nothing too drastic.

Then suddenly a force intruded that would not yield to

a cover-up. The threat of death precipitated that force. All hell seemed to break loose on my canvas and there was no way to integrate the old with what was happening. I used to think I'd rather die than act like a fool or, worse, appear unkind. I learned differently.

Actually, a few years ago I began to paint and went for some lessons. I remember my teacher telling me not to try working everything out on one canvas. Let yourself go on one, try a disciplined still life on the other. He promised me if I kept at it the two would come together.

It's been several years since my operation. I can't say that the whole "picture" has come together yet. My work with death and loss is focused primarily on a laughter group. Some of the same people who come to support group to express their grief also meet once a month for the purpose of laughing together. When you cry, your head empties, and when you laugh, it usually starts you coughing and gets some heaviness off your chest. It's good to release some of the bottled-up energy and even better to come together and share.

I had thought when I originally sat down to write this that I would discuss the therapeutic value of laughter and tears. But methods of releasing emotions, though they are helpful, are only techniques. When you go to care for someone who is dying, or you are suddenly confronted with your own death, these techniques may even get in the way.

What I've begun to realize through being on the other side of the fence is that even when you think you're not imposing your beliefs on the patient, we all have subtle expectations. We want death to be "comfortable," and most of us admire dignity in the face of disaster. But that's not always possible. The important thing to realize is that individual balance and wholeness are unique to each person.

The places each of us masks all of our lives in order to cope may, if we're lucky, be uncovered under stress, allowing us to relate to life and death in a more genuine way. But the process of unmasking can be very uncomfortable for patient and caregiver alike. In the long run, I believe, at each given moment all of us are doing the best we can do.

I don't know that I will be any better prepared when the possibility of death comes again. Yet I am deeply grateful for the opportunity to start on a fresh canvas. I like to think that each of us is working on a separate piece of a larger work, and that when we do achieve a balance and a sense of integrity, our work can be joined to the larger whole. Of course, knowing my tendency to overwork things, I suspect I'll need someone to take the paintbrushes away and say, "It's done."

Someone asked me what I had learned about forgiveness in this journey through all of the laughter and all of the tears. Well, it may seem obvious, but as the time in the hospital faded and my renewed, authentic self took over, I could use laughter (again as a healing tool) to forgive the hospital setting and the people there who had made me seem so dehumanized, so helpless, so much an object ("the mastectomy in the room down the hall"), instead of like the valuable human being, complete with anger and fears, laughter and tears, that I am.

I went through a long process of forgiving my body and forgiving the trials and tribulations that had brought me to that point in time. I had to forgive God as well. In fact, I believe that everyone—yes everyone!—has to come to a reconciliation with God. It's part of the life-affirming process. And that's where I am now. It's been five years now, and I've got a clean bill of health. I have a fresh canvas and new brushes and paint and a deep and abiding gratefulness for life.

Wants vs. Needs, or Quality of Life vs. Quality of Care

When someone you love needs more help than you can give, than anyone in the family can give, what can you do?

Usually someone who lives close by, perhaps the oldest daughter or son of an elderly parent, starts as the informal caregiver. This person checks on the parent, takes him or her to the doctor, does the shopping, pays the bills. Soon it becomes a full-time, seven-days-a-week job, especially if the caregiver does not have regular full-time work hours during which she must be elsewhere. The time spent caregiving encroaches on all other aspects of life, until the daughter is either at her father's home, on her way, reassuring him on the phone, handling his daily affairs, or all of the above. Most people have trouble doing this long-term, no matter how much they care. But they do.

It happened to me. I called myself the "daily daughter" because of my mother's increasing needs when she suffered from Parkinson's disease that turned into Alzheimer's after the first three years of her illness. I was the daily daughter because I was there, unmarried and unattached, working full-time as a writer but (to her mind at least), with no preset hours. I struggled to maintain my own boundaries and sense of self. I struggled to make a living and deal with my own grief and fatigue. I did not always succeed. I looked for other options—Meals on Wheels and Home Health Care three mornings a week. A social worker was assigned by her doctor to help our family find other solutions. My mother's condition worsened. But she was still lucid and capable of making her own decisions. She refused to have anyone come in on a full-time basis, although she longed for me to quit my own life and move into her back bedroom and take care of her. This I refused to do. I was already taking care of her, including a financial commitment that I had made five years earlier to keep a roof over her head. I got someone in to clean. I took her laundry home with me. I brought her meals at night. I took her everywhere I could, until she could no longer, even with a walker, get into my car without someone picking her up bodily. This I could not do physically.

We held family conferences. One of my sisters and her husband, who lived an hour away, became more available. One sister did not. The nearby sister and I assigned ourselves specific tasks. She and her husband would be responsible for the transportation to the doctor, the medical paperwork, and the financial paperwork involved in my mother's affairs (except for my mother's personal bills and her checkbook, which I took care of). Because my mother was soon unable to drive herself and later, unable to get in and out of my car, and because of a nagging back problem of my own, aggravated by the frequent lifting required to assist my mother's movements, my sister and her husband took over her "monthly outings." They were able at first to take her to their house for weekend visits or to see her dentist near their home.

Gradually my mother's condition worsened. She did not want to live with any of her daughters. (Although she still harbored the notion that someone should move in with her, a plan that was not feasible physically or psychologically for me.) We looked for other solutions. She was no longer able to go to a regular retirement home, due to her increasing disabilities. The condo complex she lived in was mostly retirees anyway, and served as the first step for many residents before their health failed and they needed other solutions.

I scouted the area for places with assisted living, sometimes called personal care facilities. My mother, sister, and brother-in-law came with me to visit the best of them. Again, we wanted my mother to make her own decisions for as long as possible. While money was definitely a consideration, when we added up the costs of where she was now living and the additional help she needed and would increasingly need, the choices were clear. My mother selected an attractive, well-kept, well-staffed efficiency apartment in an assisted-living building, set in a beautiful parkland close to my house. She would have three good meals a day, as well as her own kitchen in her efficiency apartment. I would no longer do the laundry or the shopping or the meals. She would have maid service and activities galore, and a special van would take those residents who were ambulatory on shopping and sightseeing trips. Someone would give her her medication and help her with daily tasks.

After a traumatic week of ten-hour days carefully and patiently sorting with my mother through her lifetime of accumulation, and designating presents to each child, grandchild, great-grandchild, and friend, we were ready to move my mother and her antique furnishings to the Courtyards. We also arranged for continuing Home Health Care aides to visit her on schedule to help her bathe and dress. A physical therapist and a Home Health Care nurse monitored her condition. I visited daily and continued to handle her increasing needs.

Alas, it wasn't enough! We had been told by the social worker that it would take at least two months, maybe longer, for my mother to adjust to her new surroundings and make friends. She was an extremely outgoing, friendly, and social woman, and one reason she had decided to move into the Courtyards was that she thought she would make friends. She was ready to be liked. She was not prepared to find that other women and men in the assisted-living building were preoccupied with their own frailties, their own illnesses, their own concerns. She told me once in bewilderment, "I thought I would be Queen of the Courtyards, but there's nothing but old, sick, selfish people here." A telling statement!

While it was a godsend to me to have a good part of my day to myself again in order to work and to put my own life back together, my mother's demands grew. Soon Home Health Care staff were seeing her seven mornings a week and other people came seven nights a week to help prepare her for bed. Nurse visits increased from once a week to daily.

Yet no matter what I did to solve the daily list of problems she presented me with, it was not enough. I realized that it would never be enough. This was a profound and unsettling change for her. Her expectations were unreasonable and unfillable. She was depressed, angry, self-pitying, needy. She wanted someone to fix her life and make everything all right. We couldn't. No one could. The staff exerted themselves in compassion and friendliness. She was urged to participate in every activity possible to her ever-increasing frailty. I took her on daily walks, ran her errands, brought special treats and meals to her. Her friends visited. Her prayer group came to meet in her room. Her family came from all over the country to visit with her and to take her places. We enlisted everyone from second cousins to grandchildren-in-law to make her place as beautiful and homey as we could.

In the space of three months, my mother moved three

times within the facility, each time needing more care. Finally she arrived at the foster care wing, right outside the aides' station, whose only criterion was that she be ambulatory (with the help of her daily and nightly helpers). More love and care was lavished on her. We thought that she had finally adjusted and was making friends, at least to talk with in the dining room, although her place had been moved from one circular table to another for several months, in order to get her to a table where she felt the people were friendly. She kept on asking people to help her. The other residents could barely help themselves, much less assist my mother. But she did make some acquaintances, although the confusion that most of the residents exhibited made for bizarre conversations. My mother's fears and nightmares increased, no matter the change of medications or change of scenery. She began to believe that certain people were trying to kill her. Her nightmares became a part of her daytime reveries as well. Each phone call from her, day or night, was an exercise in despair and fear. When I came to see her, I never knew whether she would be shaking in fright at the thought of an aide (in her mind) swinging from the shower rod to seize her and strangle her or whether she would be babbling about the children she was saving from the fire that, she was convinced, had engulfed the building. Her daytime and nighttime calls to me and to my sister became more frequent and more bizarre.

But once in a while, there she would be, a smile on her face, dressed in her beautiful clothes, her hair just done, waiting for me with open arms. We would visit and reminisce. She would be lucid, clear, the mother I remembered. But I never knew what to expect from one day to the next. The crises erupted an average of once a week; I would drop everything to go tend to whatever insurmountable problem was looming on her horizon that day. Soon these episodes increased in frequency and duration. Another resident spilled hot coffee on her lap, and she was rushed to the emergency room and then treated three times a day in her apartment by a wound care specialist, until the second-degree burns healed. An ulcer on her heel required several weeks of daily dressings and wearing special shoes. Small strokes were noted. Edema and an infection were next on the agenda.

But the hardest thing to deal with were her fears. We had originally moved her from her home because she would call the neighbors at night whenever she had nightmares. She was convinced, even then, that someone was trying to kill her. She would remain frozen in bed, convinced that her throat had been cut and that she was lying in a pool of blood, calling out for help on the phone, until a neighbor or I would arrive. We thought she would feel safer in the assisted-living facility, where my sister and I insisted that the night helper check on her personally every two hours. But her fears increased. Even though we changed her medication several times, she worsened. It was now clear that something other than the medication she was taking to control her Parkinson's disease was causing the hallucinations. I knew she had Alzheimer's, although no one else in the family, at that time, wanted to admit it. It was clear to me and to everyone else that something had to be done. But we continued to assist her where she was, hoping that another move would not be necessary. We did not want to destroy her already tenuous hold on reality.

One morning my mother, standing at the antique buffet in her room, not three steps from her wicker armchair, where she had been sitting watching TV, turned her body slightly to look out the double windows that fronted on parkland. She liked to watch the birds outside on the patio. In that brief instant she lost her balance and fell, cracking three ribs and cutting her head open as she fell on her glasses. As she was rushed to the emergency room by ambulance, I knew that a corner had been turned. She could no longer be considered ambulatory in any sense of the word. She would have to be moved into a skilled nursing facility. The piecemeal efforts we had made for the last three years at providing Mother with the best possible quality of life, considering her deteriorating physical and mental condition, were at an end.

After six hours in the emergency room, my mother was discharged. The hospital did not want to admit her, since it would take weeks, perhaps months, for her ribs to heal. She could not go back to the assisted-living facility. She could not go to my sister's house. Although we were prepared for eventual nursing home care, and had visited several and tentatively made arrangements for that eventuality, all the places on our list were full. It was late Friday afternoon. Frantic calls and paperwork ensued. Meanwhile, my mother lay immobile, bemused, waiting for the next ambulance ride. The seventeen stiches in her head near her eyes plus the huge shiner she sported around one eye gave her the appearance of a defeated prizefighter, down for the count. Finally, late Friday night, my sister and I were able to find a facility that would accept her. My mother's eyes lit up when she heard. "I'm going there," she gasped. "Oh, I've always wanted to live there." "There" was the Cadillac of nursing homes and retirement homes, clustered around a skilled nursing health center.

After my mother had taken her second ambulance ride of the day, this from the hospital to the skilled nursing facility, and my sister and I had completed all the paperwork at the health center, we went upstairs to her new room to see how my mother was.

She was holding court. Clustered around her bed were the director of the facility, the head nurse, the heads of physical, speech, and occupational therapy, a young aide who had been assigned to her, and the floor nurse. Yes, it was a skilled nursing unit in a nursing home. Yes, she had to share a room. Yes, even the comfort of the place and the tender loving care the staff showed could not disguise the fact that it was an institutional setting. But this was as good as it got.

In the space of nine months we had moved my mother five times (not counting two trips to the hospital emergency room). We did not know then that there would be other falls, other broken bones, other trips to the hospital, extensive and expensive and continuing physical, occupational, and speech therapy, and eventually, even more moves within the same facility. Perhaps it was better that we did not know.

We did realize one important insight, one that every caregiver and family member should know. We had shifted our emphasis from quality of life—all that we could do for Mother for her to have the best life possible—to quality of care.

This is an important distinction. A friend told me, and this was echoed by the director of the assisted-living facility, that when a person begins to need caregiving beyond the normal everyday help that family and friends are willing to provide, the person and the family must go from attending to only the *wants* of the person to addressing primarily his or her *needs*. I remember the director of the assisted-living facility, where my mother first lived, saying in a bemused tone of voice, "Well, Helen was always such an interesting puzzle, such a unique challenge to us to meet her wants and needs." That was as tactful as she could get!

My sister and I realized that we had gone from doing all that we could to fulfill my mother's wants, which centered around living independently in her own home forever, to trying to meet her needs, which included the three moves within the assisted-living facility, each one a step closer to more care and less autonomy. We had arrived at a stage in my mother's life journey in which we had to shift our main consideration from quality of life issues to quality of care ones.

So we moved her for the final time (we hoped). Of course we surrounded her bed by the window with her favorite books and family photographs, her television and VCR; she had her music, her brightly colored handmade quilt on the bed, her special pillows, her personal effects, her favorite clothes. But it was still a skilled nursing facility. Certainly one of the best available, with physical therapy, speech therapy, occupational therapy, a choice of activities as permitted, good meals, unlimited visiting hours, and visiting areas that were more beautiful and well kept than the average home. Nonetheless, it was an institution.

I would like to say that my mother, once it was explained to her that her ribs would take time to heal, accepted the change in her circumstances with good grace. She did, initially, loving her therapy, making friends with the nurses and aides, tolerating her first roommate, a difficult and confused woman. But after a week or two of the newness, my mother became disoriented. Before, she had been lucid 70 percent of the time, and confused and hallucinatory about 30 percent of the time. Now the percentages flipped. Increasingly she was in another world. Sometimes she greeted me with the assertion that she had died, although she told me, looking around critically, "It's not near as nice a place as I thought it would be. I really expected Heaven." Other times she insisted that she was in jail and that the nurses were torturing her and keeping her confined against her will.

Sometimes she would think that she was in London, or out in the country, and increasingly, on trains going somewhere, anywhere, lost in whatever decade she had previously lived in. "I can get as far as London," she told me one day as I left, "but I can't quite get to heaven."

Then my mother fell again, this time while pulling out the drawer of her bedside table. And then again. And yet again. This, despite the fact that each time she was helped out of bed she was now accompanied by either myself or at least one aide, sometimes two. Old fractures were rebroken. Another round of physical therapy ensued. Each day that I visited, I never knew whether she would be "there" or not. Sometimes it took an hour of talking to bring her back into the present. Sometimes nothing helped.

Yet there were still times, increasingly rare, when she awaited me with a sweet smile, her eyes clear. "There's my darling daughter," she would exclaim. "Let's go on a trip." A trip being downstairs and out the front to sit on the breezeway at the entrance. Or up and down the elevators to the various lounges on the various floors, to see what was happening in the areas where the retirees and the assisted-living residents lived. I never knew what to expect, whether to get a wheelchair, her walker, or call for a nurse.

One morning, while holding on to her walker, with one aide in front of her and one aide holding on to her back, she slid down between them. Her right hip broke in two places. The doctor told us that sometimes the hip crumbles and then the person falls, rather than the hip shattering on impact with the floor. My mother was in the hospital for seven days, with major surgery the first day. My sister and I kept vigil, taking shifts at the hospital. My mother's incoherency, anger, frustration, and depression increased. She would babble for hours and then turn on me in swift anger. Once when I had stayed for ten hours straight then gone home to get some sleep, she accused me when I returned of abandoning her for days. She was like an animal with its leg caught in a trap. She cried out in fear whenever she was turned in bed. When the nurse explained that she was only moving her bad leg, my mother cried, "My leg isn't bad. It's an innocent leg. Don't hurt it."

After a week in the hospital it was determined that my mother would not be able to undertake the level of intensive rehab that the hospital provided. She was moved back to her nursing home to the rehab floor there. Her nurses, aides, and therapists welcomed her to a new room with a beautiful view, just across from the physical therapy station. They hugged her and kissed her and assured her that she would get better. Yet even the first day back, after the therapists had assessed her condition, we knew that my mother would never walk again. And her increasing mental confusion made it difficult for her to carry through on relearning and remembering the simplest tasks. "It will be too demoralizing for her to be in this wing for twenty-one days and then have to move again to another wing when she is no longer eligible for therapy due to her prognosis," they told my sister and me. "Better to move her now, at once, today, so that she won't have yet another adjustment to make."

So my mother was moved to another room, down a long hall that did not advertise, and yet we knew, that this was the quiet wing, the bedridden wing, the last wing. Her therapists would come to her for whatever limited rehab she could do. They would come to her and turn her and lift

her and get her in and out of the wheelchair so that she
would not remain immobile. They would attempt speech
therapy and occupational therapy as well as physical therapy, all of which my mother looked forward to eagerly
when she was lucid. But even the most optimistic among
us knew that even as her bones were crumbling, so too was
her brain stem disintegrating. My mother had now been
moved eight times in a little over a year. We continued
with whatever physical, occupational, and speech therapy
she could manage. But it was short-term. Nothing could
stem the tide of my mother's decreasing strength and coherency. All the love and care in the world could not re-
verse her physical, mental, and emotional disintegration.

It is hard when the child becomes the parent and the
parent becomes the child. It is hard to let go of the person
you love so dearly and let her hold on to you at the same
time. I kept looking around, the first year or so that my
mother was ill, for someone to help me with this enormous
task I had been given. I had promised to be there for her.
I had promised to see her through. It was a constant, fa-
tiguing, and enormous task, an unending spiritual test, to
keep that promise.

I wanted to talk to someone, to share my pain. Since my
mother had always been there for me, had always been
there for others in the family when illnesses and deaths occurred, I looked to the one person who could help me
cope with this daily loss I was experiencing. But she *was*
the daily loss. More than undergoing this reversal in our
positions, I had lost my rock in a storm. I had lost my
cheerful, busy, independent, loving mother. I lost her inch
by inch, day by day, year by year.

It was useless to say, "Let go," when she was holding on
for dear life. Useless to say, "Don't care. Steel yourself,"

when everything within me cried out for her loving arms, her strength, her practical advice.

She had taught me well. Be strong. Care for others. Love and love and love again no matter what. But who would comfort me? Who can comfort me? No one, never again. Sometimes I feel like a motherless child, but I am the mother now. I am the mother and the caregiver and the project manager and the decision maker. I am the sustenance to this dying lady.

I don't want her to suffer anymore. I don't want to suffer anymore. I see death as a kind friend in this situation. And death is overdue. Death is dragging her feet. Death is late.

I squeeze my mother's hand and kiss her good-bye each day and I tell her softly, "I'll love you forever." She smiles, she knows. "Love you forever too," she whispers when she can, when her mind clears for even a few moments. This is the truth about us no matter the terrible times that are happening now. No matter the agony of being the witness to her travail. And yet. And yet. I need my mother. I want my mother. Now, above all, I need her loving arms to help me through.

Responsibility and Caregiving

Diane Harvey is the health education director of a renowned hospital and holds a Ph.D. as well as a degree in nursing. I originally wanted to interview her because of the programs she offers, including an Alzheimer's support group. But as we drove together to a conference I was to address, she shared with me, instead, her own personal story of caregiving.

My mother has Alzheimer's disease. Despite other siblings, I ended up as the primary caregiver. Sound familiar? I've heard this again and again in the caregiver support groups. My mother is a lovely, intelligent lady, and we were very close. I say "were" because her whole personality has changed since her disease worsened.

I love my mother dearly, and as a nurse, I know she cannot control what is happening to her brain. But as a daughter, oh my! I have struggled with so many tears and set and reset boundaries and made promises to myself that I would—must—have a life of my own.

I am a single parent with a son and a daughter and I hold an interesting and demanding job with lots of responsibility. When I looked at my life in the context of my mother's illness, I saw that there was not anything I could give up in order to spend more and more time to care for my mother, no matter her demands. I just couldn't meet everyone's needs, no matter how hard I tried.

I've always been told that I am the responsible one in the family. I just do my best, and stamina and a good sense of humor usually get me through. But one week— Well, I can tell you that it was truly the week from hell!

First my St. Bernard gave birth to seven puppies on my bed! Then my teenage son got into trouble and really needed me. His distress at the continuing demands on my time with the added caregiver responsibility was evident. Then my mother fell and fractured her hip, and was rushed to the hospital. My young daughter accompanied me during our visits to the hospital, and we would often arrive home exhausted at the end of a long, tiring day that often stretched into the late evening hours.

One night we had just rolled into the driveway from our nightly visit to my mother. It was about 8:30 P.M. and we had not eaten. I just wanted to fix a quick supper and sit down with my daughter. The phone rang. It was the hospital. My mother had gone into an uncontrollable rage and was violent. No one could do anything with her. The nurse on duty urged me to return as soon as possible.

"I'll be there in fifteen minutes," I promised. My daughter was listening and watching me. I leaned against the stove and burst into tears. It was all too much for me.

My daughter was crying too. "Mom," she said. "Couldn't we please have supper first? Surely you're allowed to have supper. We need our supper, Mom." She took me by the hand. "Ever since I've known you," she said, solemn as a judge, like an adult talking to a crying child, "you've been responsible. Couldn't you please, please, please, just this once, *not* be responsible?"

Her words hit home. I stopped crying. I picked up the phone and called the hospital again. I spoke to the charge nurse. "I'll be a little late," I said. "You'll have to handle her until I get there. It will probably be about forty minutes or so. Yes. I'm going to have supper with my daughter first. Yes. It's up to you."

From that moment on I knew I would have to set my priorities and stick to them, no matter how difficult it was for both my mother and me emotionally. There were other people who needed me as well. And I didn't always have to be responsible.

My mother doesn't understand. She will never be able to understand. But I cannot meet all her needs and mine as well. I remember her as she was, and I honor her as my mother. But I find I have to pull away more and more, or else I am sucked into that terrible maelstrom of anger and fear and need that rules her life now. I am gentle with her. But I am more gentle with myself as well. And every time it seems hopeless and exhausting, I whisper to myself, "You don't always have to be responsible. You can take a break. You can let go of this for a little while. You can have a normal supper with your daughter." And that helps me to keep my sanity.

More and More Guilt

I thought I had resolved all guilt, both real and false, laid on me both by myself and by my mother, during the first two years of my mother's illness. I couldn't even remember what it was I felt guilty about, unless it was the on-going theme of not being able to meet my mother's wants, needs, expectations, and desires. I was doing what I could. It had to be enough.

I tried my best neither to judge my mother nor to allow myself to be manipulated by her, a tiring and frustrating task that many caregivers face, especially mothers and daughters. I just wanted to continue helping and loving my mother.

I'll never forget one pivotal day, when in the midst of horrendous double book deadlines, after phone calls and reassurances to the nurses and to my mother that I would visit her that afternoon (as I did daily), the front desk on the skilled nursing floor at the health care center called me one more time. "Your mother has barricaded herself behind her chairs and bed," they announced. "She is out of control, angry, and fearful. We've tried reasoning with her, but she will only talk to you. We don't want to frighten her, or tackle her. We're afraid of hurting her fragile bones. We can't get close enough to sedate her. Please come now! We can do nothing!"

So I went. In despair, anger, frustration I went. If it had been anyone but my mother, standing there with chairs pushed in front of her five-foot tall, less than a hundred pound body, I would, perhaps, have found the situation ludicrous. Here was an elderly woman, increasingly out of her mind, with cracked ribs and edema and infections and Parkinson's and Alzheimer's and ulcers, holding an entire hospital wing at bay. Insisting that her daughter be there. Controlling us all.

I walked in and put my arms around her and guided her to the bed, where we sat with me holding her while the attendants rearranged the room and tiptoed out for her medicine. After soothing my mother down, I asked her what was wrong and what I could do to help. I did not know what kind of answer I would get. Sometimes she was set off by the way someone had looked at her while helping her to dress, or the wrong food at breakfast, or being hurried, or her roommate, or her boredom. Sometimes it was the therapists, and what they demanded of her. Sometimes it was the TV, which we usually turned off because she tended to get overly stimulated and "go into the picture" and live whatever was happening on TV. So I held her and soothed her and waited for her to tell me what was wrong.

My mother then became perfectly lucid, or at least according to her reasoning. She wanted to see me right now, she explained, because she had thought long and hard about who was going to die with her. She had decided that since my other two sisters had husbands, she had decided that I was going to die with her.

My anger turned to despair. I felt like someone had kicked me in the stomach. I tried to reason with her. "Mama, I'm not going to die with you. I have many more years to live, as I am younger than you. I have too much work to do!" What a bizarre conversation!

"But you must," she insisted. "You're the only one who loves me. If you love me you'll die with me. I'm afraid to go alone. I want you to keep me company." Again and again I tried to reason with her, in this increasingly strange and sorrowful conversation. It was like pitting myself against a steel door.

"No, Mama, I'm not going to die with you. It's not my time. This is something you need to talk over with God. It's not up to me to die with you." I tried to steady my voice through my tears.

My mother drew away from me angrily. "You're not in good health," she cried. "And you're all alone. You have to come with me." She delivered the final blow. "If you don't die with me, you'll always feel guilty."

That broke the spell. "Why would I feel guilty, Mama?" I asked her quietly.

"Because you're an ungrateful daughter," she announced. The words fell between us on the bed. I drew a deep breath.

"I have nothing to feel guilty about, Mama," I said quietly, still holding on to her, still trying to get through to her with my love, the love that was there behind the despair, looking into her eyes, praying that she would understand me. "You know how much I love you, but I will *not* die with you and for you. I know that I am a good daughter. I have nothing to reproach myself for. I'm not guilty of anything, Mama, and you cannot make me feel guilty, no matter what you say."

My mother started crying. She peeked through her fingers covering her eyes, to see what effect this was having on me. "Oh poor, poor me," she gasped. "To have to go through this alone. You'll be sorry."

The nurse came in with her tranquilizer. We laid my mother back on her bed. I fled the room.

It took me some time to deal with my feelings of anger and betrayal. But I did. It taught me a valuable lesson in love and in caregiving. I now refuse to feel guilty over anything concerning my mother's care. When I am overly tired and the despair comes creeping in and I feel that her travail will never end, I look in the mirror and say to myself, "Not guilty."

The Dream That Changed My Father's Life

Not all caregiver stories are ones of despair. No matter the daily intensity and the eventual outcome, much of caregiving is rewarding and worthwhile. Sometimes there is even joy. Mary Schramski, a beautiful and intelligent writer friend of mine, told me the story of her father and the caregiving journey they shared.

In November of 1991, the doctors told me and my father, Jim Hauser, that he was dying. My father was a seventy-two-year-old former airline pilot, seemingly fit, healthy, energetic. Now he had a malignant tumor on his spine. According to the doctors, his prognosis was problematic. They predicted he had only a few months to live and prescribed radiation treatments and painkillers.

I had spent most of my life separated from my father. I did not know him very well. But I did know that he had never been sick a day in his life and that he had been careful with his nutrition and exercise. For many years he had run ten miles a day. As he grew older he reduced his exercise to miles of daily walking.

I resolved to spend as much time with my father as I could. These were the last days of his life. I resigned my job as a college teacher and I traveled back and forth between Keller, Texas, where I lived, and my father's home in

Las Cruces, New Mexico. I was with him all during the radiation treatments, and I personally monitored his daily medication.

My father's condition worsened. By early January he refused to eat, would not get out of bed, and was deeply depressed. He weighed only about one hundred pounds. His body was emaciated. He had lost all hope and had no interest in anything or anyone. I believed at that time he was ready to die, and I steeled myself for that event.

But then I decided to take him home with me to Texas. I wanted my father to die in my home. His doctors protested that he was too weak to make the trip, but I insisted.

I resolved to do two things during my father's last days. I would make him as comfortable as possible and I would do everything in my power to get to know as much about my father as I could. I spent most of each day with him. We talked in ever-increasing intimacy.

We spent some time together outdoors every day. I took him for drives. I found things for him to do. But mostly we talked. We shared a lifetime as we talked.

Then I altered the medication plan that the doctors had prescribed. Instead of giving my father a handful of painkillers and tranquilizers every two hours, I waited until he asked for them. His requests came farther and farther apart. Amazingly, he began to feel better. He started spending more time out of bed. He went three days without any pain medication. He could not get enough of his conversations with me. We looked forward each day to our talks. He became more alert and interested in life. Then he began to speak of the future. I made him have hope.

My father did not die in 1992. He went back to his walking, developed a hearty appetite, and began a program of nutrition. He returned to Las Cruces and sold his property there. He then returned to Keller, bought a lot, and built a home for himself in order to be close to me and my husband. We are still getting to know and love one another.

No one in the medical field can explain what happened to my father. I think that my father was dying because he did not care about living, and something happened to give him hope and a reason to live. Hope and purpose encouraged his brain and his body. His brain began to send messages of living instead of messages of dying to his body. My father decided at that time to live joyfully.

There is an interesting postscript to my father's remarkable recovery. Near the end of his recuperation in my home, my father told me about the following dream he had one night.

He dreamed that he was a passenger on an airplane, sitting at the back of the plane instead of flying the plane as he had in real life. The plane was flying low over a large city and at times it sank down into the valleys between the looming skyscrapers. The plane banked and turned and flew in a dangerous but exhilarating manner. It was an exciting, soaring flight. Despite having flown aiplanes for thirty-six years, my father then became overwhelmed with fear as the plane turned again and again. He decided to go up to the cockpit to see who the captain was. When he opened the door to the cockpit, he was surprised to see that the captain was his deceased older brother, Gray. He had admired and loved this brother all of his life.

Seeing him standing there in the doorway, his brother Gray said to him, "Jim, you go back to your seat and relax. I'll fly this flight for you."

My father realized then that this was not the flight on which he was supposed to die. That he had more time. He explained to me that he felt that his older brother was there to lead and encourage and inspire him.

Mary ended her story by saying that she felt the power in her father's dream and in his telling of the dream. That she felt that her father had tapped into a human experience that many of us do not recognize when we are on the ground. That all of our older brothers and sisters who have gone before us into death are there to lead and encourage and inspire us, just as his brother did. Her father told Mary that after the dream, he felt that he could relax and enjoy the flight. For however long it might be. And that he was at peace about the rest of his journey.

Practical Aspects of Caregiving

Excerpted from the "1995 Guide to Health Insurance for People with Medicare."

There are some hard truths about the practical aspects of caregiving. But fortunately there is help available of many kinds. Finding your way through the maze of options available as the informal caregiving turns into a full-time responsibility is the crux of the matter. Here are guidelines from the latest information on Medicare and long-term care options. The resource guide in the back of this book will lead you to telephone numbers of agencies you can call to obtain specific information in your area for your specific needs.

WHAT IS LONG-TERM CARE?

Long-term care is increasingly becoming a predictable life event for a large part of the population.

You'll often see nursing home care referred to as long-term care. However, long-term care (LTC) refers to a broad range of medical, personal and environmental services designed to assist individuals who have lost the ability to remain completely independent in the community. Nursing home care is only one aspect of a full span of services included in the definition of long-term care. There are three major categories of long-term care: institutional care, home health care, and community based care.

THE NEED FOR LONG-TERM CARE

Typically, the need for long-term care arises when physical or mental conditions impair a person's ability to perform at least some of the basic activities of everyday life. These include: eating, toileting (ability to control the toileting process), continence (bladder and bowel control), bathing, dressing, ambulating (ability to move oneself) and transferring (ability to travel without assistance). Long-term care may be provided by family, friends or a number of health care professionals. Professional care is generally divided into three levels:

1. **Skilled care.** Continuous around-the-clock care provided by licensed medical professionals under the direct supervision of a physician. For practical reasons this level of care is usually provided in an institutional setting such as a skilled nursing facility.

2. **Intermediate care.** Intermittent care provided by registered nurses (RNs), licensed practical nurses (LPNs) and nurse's aides under the supervision of a physician. While this level of care may be provided in the home it is more practical when provided in an institutional setting.

3. **Custodial care.** Assistance in meeting activities of daily living provided by a number of professional and non-professional caregivers under the supervision of a physician. This level of care may be provided in any of the long-term care sources.

TYPES OF LONG-TERM CARE SERVICES

Long-term care services are designed to assist individuals who need care because of a prolonged illness, surgery or disability. Care may be provided by informal caregivers (immediate family, relatives or friends), as well as formal or professional providers (physicians, nurses and therapists) and community-based service providers (adult day-care and senior centers). Care can range from chore types of services to around-the-clock skilled nursing care. Formal care becomes necessary when family caregiving is inadequate or inappropriate.

As individuals age, they are likely to suffer from acute and/or chronic illnesses or conditions. An acute illness is a serious condition, such as pneumonia or influenza, from which the body may fully recover with proper medical attention. The patient may need some assistance with chores for short periods of time until recovery and rehabilitation from the illness is complete.

Some people will suffer from chronic conditions—such as arthritis, heart disease or hypertension—that are treatable but not curable illnesses. When chronic conditions such as diabetes or heart disease initially manifest, many people ignore the inconvenience or pain they cause. Over time, however, a chronic condition frequently goes beyond being a nuisance and begins to inhibit a person's independence. Eventually he or she must look to others for help with various activities such as eating, bathing or dressing. Many people with chronic illnesses eventually become disabled and need long-term care.

Because of chronic conditions or illnesses, the elderly or disabled often suffer from limitations in performing activities that most people take for granted. These activities of daily living (ADLs), include ambulating, eating, dressing, toileting, continence, bathing and transferring from one location to another. The elderly may also be limited in performing one or more instrumental activities of daily living (IADLs), such as completing housework, using the telephone, managing money or preparing meals.

A person's loss of independence tends to occur in a predictable order. The first sign of a mental or physical impairment is usually demonstrated by a person's inability to handle simple IADLs. Then walking becomes more difficult, making a telephone call may be confusing or paying bills on time may be an impossible task for an elderly person. Generally, a walker or wheelchair will solve the problem of movement and a family member or friend can make telephone calls or pay bills.

Over time, the elderly person may also find that ADLs also become difficult to complete. At this point, needed care can be scheduled. For example, a family member might bathe and dress the individual in the morning. After work, he or she may return to assist the impaired person with dressing for bed. Such a routine can be effective for people who need relatively little assistance. However, people who need assistance with toileting or transferring cannot wait for that assistance; it must be delivered on demand. Regular, full-time assistance is needed at this point.

When an impaired person suffers some physical or mental impairment, care is often initially provided by family members or friends. However, some people have no available family or friend caregivers. Professionals are also needed when families are no longer able or willing to provide needed care. That reality, along with a general increase in the incidence of chronic illness, has produced an enormous need for people who can supply medical, environmental and personal care to the elderly.

Medical Care. After surgery, or as the result of an accident or illness, an elderly person may need medical care. Such care may help maintain the person's health status, slow the progress of the condition that restricts the individual's independence or promote recuperation from a hospital stay or surgery. This care is typically provided by a registered nurse (RN), a licensed practical nurse (LPN) or another type of health-care professional in an institutional, community or home setting. Advances in medical science have made the delivery of health-related care in the home easier and more efficient.

Typically, medical care is needed because of an acute condition that inhibits one's physical abilities. Individuals with these conditions will either recover, be rehabilitated or die. Medical long-term care will last for shorter periods of time than either environmental or personal care.

Environmental Care. Activities that a healthy person takes for granted, such as grocery shopping, housecleaning and paying bills, present huge difficulties for the ill or disabled person. These are daily tasks to assure that the household operates smoothly; they range from basic housekeeping to balancing a checkbook.

When a person is disabled, the environment in which he or she lives can become threatening rather than comforting. Stairways, basements and long hallways become physical barriers. Labor-saving devices such as microwave ovens or remote controls may be confusing to operate. Simple chores that once took only a small part of a day, such as preparing a meal or washing clothes, now take hours to complete.

In most cases, an elderly or a disabled person's family or friends are called on to provide environmental care. They may provide yard maintenance and exterior repairs, such as painting and roof repair. In addition to cleaning the home, they may adapt the interior with grab bars in the bathroom, or widen doorways to accommodate a wheelchair or install ramps to suit the disabled person's needs.

Personal Care. Like environmental care, personal care is designed to help the elderly or disabled person throughout the day with tasks that healthy people take for granted. These include bathing, dressing, toileting, transferring from a bed or chair and eating. The amount of assistance required varies by the level of disability or impairment that exists. Some people need help for every activity of daily living; others need only minor assistance; some simply need a reminder to complete a task.

Such simple activities as using a telephone, driving an automobile, using public transportation, or handling money can also be considered personal care. Again, the assistance required will depend on the degree of the person's disability. In addition to family assistance, some communities also offer supportive or social services such as senior centers, telephone reassurance programs, church activities and Meals-on-Wheels programs.

Nursing Homes

FORMAL CARE IN A FACILITY

At some point, it's possible a care recipient will need care twenty-four hours a day. When this happens, the family caregiver becomes a project manager at home who coordinates nursing care, family visits, personal care, feeding and so on. It is at this point that most care recipients will be best served in a facility by professional caregivers.

Retired or elderly people do not necessarily wish to remain in the family home. Although their health may be excellent, they may be less interested in yard work or housekeeping than they once were. Or, they may have some medical problems that are not yet severe enough to require medical assistance. Yet many seniors enjoy their independence and prefer to remain on their own as long as possible. There are several viable options for these elderly people.

BOARD-AND-CARE HOMES

Not everyone who requires some measure of long-term care is an elderly citizen. Physically and mentally handicapped citizens often need long-term care from formal caregivers. Special facilities known as board-and-care homes are licensed by the state to provide living and care arrangements for people with special needs who are otherwise capable and anxious to live in the community. These homes offer a friendly environment, meals and some personal care under the supervision of trained individuals.

Board-and-care homes usually provide the residents with individual rooms and bathroom facilities, meals, laundry services and housekeeping services. Although residents may come and go as they please, transportation to shopping centers or social events is often provided by the home. In addition, staff members offer assistance with personal care, such as dressing and bathing, for an additional fee.

These homes are usually operated by private enterprises and the quality of care and services varies widely. The cost of board-and-care homes also varies depending on the services. Licensing requirements do not guarantee acceptable facilities: a few homes fail to comply with fire codes, sanitary conditions or inspection recommendations. However, the vast majority provide care in accordance with their license.

RESIDENTIAL CARE FACILITIES FOR THE ELDERLY

Residential care facilities for the elderly (RCFEs) provide residents with their own individual apartments. These facilities are most appropriate for seniors who wish to maintain their privacy while taking advantage of several support services that a community setting can provide. Most of these facilities offer prepared meals in a central dining room, housekeeping and laundry services, transportation for shopping, planned social activities and preventive health services, such as blood pressure checks and assistance with medications. Normally a nurse is on call for residents who need limited amounts of health care. Long-term care insurance policies that offer "assisted living" benefits may only provide this coverage when it is given through a RCFE, but only as long as the RCFE is licensed to provide such care.

Residential care facilities vary greatly in size, from those able to house five individuals to those that have adequate space to accommodate 250 people or more. The costs for assisted-living facilities vary widely, depending on the size of the facility and the amenities offered.

CONTINUING CARE RETIREMENT COMMUNITIES

Continuing care retirement communities (CCRCs) or life care communities offer a combination of informal and formal care. Generally, these facilities are intended to provide residents, who are fairly independent, with some assistance in making meals or taking medications. Residents may live in the facility for a definite or indefinite period of time. But, because the facility is prepared to meet residents' needs if they become more disabled and need skilled nursing care, the residents are afforded peace of mind. They know they will be appropriately cared for in the same community as they age.

All CCRCs will offer an area for independent living for residents still able to care for themselves and a nursing facility for residents in need of assistance. As residents lose their ability to remain independent, they can move from the independent area to the nursing area as the condition worsens. In addition, CCRCs guarantee access to quality care as an individual's needs change.

The financial arrangements vary by facility. The most common funding method requires an initial lump-sum payment followed by a monthly maintenance charge. This upfront payment can be as much as $100,000 or more for an individual. In most cases, residents pay for additional health care and nursing home services they may need in one of three ways:

1. Charges for care are included in the regular monthly bill, even if the services are not used.
2. The regular monthly bill subsidizes needed care, but residents must pay the balance of the charges.
3. The full cost of the care is billed separately from monthly maintenance charges.

NURSING HOMES

Individuals who require professional around-the-clock medical care will usually enter a skilled nursing facility or nursing home. In fact, one out of every five elderly persons who has lost the ability to remain independent is currently residing in a nursing home; the others are receiving care from one of the other providers discussed earlier.

People enter nursing homes for a number of reasons. The most common reason is that they need more care than another household or family member can, or is willing to, provide. Other commonly cited reasons for entering a nursing home include: problems completing everyday activities, no one at home to provide the care, not enough money to purchase care at home, and recuperation from surgery or illness.

Nursing homes provide around-the-clock medical care, often to patients recently discharged from a hospital. They treat people with complex nursing and rehabilitative needs, such as intravenous therapy or physical therapy. In theory, the goal of every skilled nursing facility is to rehabilitate the patient so that he or she can return home. In practice, however, a lack of care alternatives can mean that the patient will be transferred to an intermediate or custodial care unit in the same facility.

Statistically, the majority of those entering nursing homes received care in either another nursing home or a hospital while just over one-third came from a residence. The majority of people initially entering nursing homes are there for less than one year and are discharged either back home or to a hospital, or they die. Although one-third of nursing home residents remain in the facility for one year or less, the average stay is two and a half years. One-third have been there between one and three years and one-third have been in the facility three or more years. Considering that the average skilled nursing facility costs over $40,000 per year (depending on location and services

from a heart attack may need someone to help with daily tasks.

Deciding to care for a disabled or ill elderly person represents a commitment to quality care and to preserving that person's dignity and health. It is not an easy task to become an informal caregiver; it takes great emotional and physical stamina. When people care for loved ones at home, there is little relief for the caregiver. Fortunately, many communities offer a variety of options—from Meals-on-Wheels programs to senior centers—to allow the caregiver to escape the worries and frustrations of long-term care for a few minutes or a few hours. And, when the need for care exceeds the abilities of the informal caregiver or community, it is reassuring to know that home health agencies and skilled nursing facilities generally provide better quality care today than at any time in the past.

Lessons I Have Learned from Other Caregivers

Set boundaries. This is the best advice I ever got, and I was reluctant to follow it. I thought that "unconditionally" meant that you gave of yourself all the time, every hour of the day or night, no matter what. I learned that I must set limits on myself, and set loving limits on what other people could expect from me. Otherwise, there would be nothing left in me to give. Love may often feel like sacrifice, but it doesn't have to mean sacrifice. If you don't take care of yourself, there will be no one to take care of the person you are caring for. And there will be no one to take care of you.

Keep a part of your life for yourself. This means that you deserve privacy, which helps give you a chance to process and deal with your emotions. You deserve to have a part of your life—whether it is in your career, your friendships, exercising, being with others, or being alone—in which you lay aside the burden of caregiving at least for a little while, and just be yourself.

You are more than a caregiver. This label does not define you. Your purpose in this life is broader than to achieve anyone else's expectations or approval. Be true to yourself.

You will never, never, never be able to meet all of your loved one's needs, wants, wishes, and expectations. It is a futile task. Do what you can. Share the load as best you can. Your loved one may need to learn limits as well.

Honor your emotions. We have all been taught to honor our parents. We cherish and honor and respect the one we are caring for. We show our love daily, in so many ways. Isn't it also just as important to honor our own feelings? Sometimes we are going to be impatient or frustrated or angry or bone-weary or so very sad we can hardly serve another. At that time we must replenish ourselves. Like children, we must have a "time out" to sort ourselves out and rebalance. Take the time, no matter how hard it is to say no to your loved one.

Look for the lesson in the middle of the challenge. It is said that God never gives us more than we can handle. I am not sure that a long-time caregiver would agree with that statement. To gain perspective on the situation, take a step back and reflect often on the lessons you are learning. Are you learning patience? Diplomacy? Are you learning to be more loving? To communicate better? Are you experiencing such a depth of emotions that you will never be the same again? Are you gaining compassion? Clarity? Stamina? Are you learning time and energy organization? Give thanks for all that you are learning, even in the midst of the pain.

Don't let anyone else decide what you must do or not do for your loved one. You know the situation better than anyone else. You know your loved one's personality. You know your own character, your own physical limitations. Maybe another person would have moved her loved one into her home for five years. Maybe another person would have hired a home care companion. Maybe another person would have kept her job. Maybe another person would have found a way, any way, to do it differently. They are not you.

Sometimes there are no solutions. You just do the best you can, one day at a time, and only much later can you look back and say "I did it. I have nothing to reproach myself for. I was there."

Encourage the rest of the family to help you. Some won't. Some will. It still won't be enough. But you are not their conscience. You can't coerce them into helping you or your loved one. Resentment over the lack of load-sharing takes up valuable time and energy that you need for yourself. Keep on doing what you feel is right. Others may or may not help. Life is neither fair nor equal. You, at least, will know that you have done your best.

Give up any preconceived ideas about how people are supposed to behave when they are ill, or how or when they are supposed to die. The soul has its own agenda. You're not in charge of your loved one's feelings. You can't spare them. You can't bear their pain (although it often feels as if you are doing just that!). Most people come to an acceptance in their own way and in their own time. Some will fight to the last breath! The process cannot be rushed or hurried. Exhortations about "going to the light" may only inspire our loved ones to think that we want to get rid of them, when they are not yet ready to go. The opposite is true as well.

You cannot hold on to your loved one when he or she is ready to go. Don't hang on. Let go. Little by little, you too must come to an acceptance of the situation.

To prolong a life unduly, when the person you love is suffering so, is unkind. To beg the person to get well is even more unkind. To praise him for getting better, to show your disappointment and impatience when he doesn't, is both cruel and unkind. I once knew a couple who, in their zeal to help their elderly father and because of their own unexpressed fear of death, stuffed their loved one with so many nutrients (seventeen supplements a day!) that the poor man could neither assimilate nor even swallow them all. Perhaps the supplements, in moderation, could have helped at an earlier stage of the man's illness. But he was both mentally and physically impaired, and had suffered through a long, debilitating illness. Your loved one will not meet your expectations of either living longer, getting well, or dying with a smile. One of the strongest lessons of caregiving is learning to give up control over another human being's life. Let it be.

It's okay to feel both relief and sadness when your loved one lets go. Grief takes a long time. If it has been a long illness and especially if you have been the primary caregiver, physical exhaustion and emotional overload have already taken their toll. You need rest and recuperation. Nature has an interesting way of shutting down the receptors in the brain when you are on overload. Some people experience this as a merciful numbness right after their loved one has died. This carries you through the first few days or weeks until you are strong enough to deal with your loss.

If the person you have cared for is elderly and has lingered for a long time, there can be an added element of relief and acceptance. Surely you don't want your loved one to suffer anymore. It's okay for you to feel whatever you feel after the death of a loved one. It's time to let go and heal.

Don't let anyone tell you how to mourn, or how long to mourn, or to dictate your feelings in any way. You have been through a long and tiring journey of giving and learning and caring and loving. Now is your time. Don't rush the mourning process or the recuperative process.

There is life after caregiving. You will find your way back in your own time and on your own terms.

Some people feel guilty for living when their loved one has died. This is called "survivor's guilt." It's okay for you to go on. It's okay for you to find joy and meaning in your life again. You are alive! And your life is valuable and precious. Give yourself permission to get on with it. You deserve happiness.

Family Possessions

I originally wrote this for A Soulworker's Companion
*and it is reprinted here with the generous permission
of Wildcat Canyon Press.*

My mother moved five times in one year, from her home into an assisted-living community, where she changed rooms with each level of increasing care, and finally onto a skilled nursing floor at another health center, her final move in this lifetime.

One of my sisters helped me move her. Again and again we moved her.

We are probably the only two sisters in the Western Hemisphere who didn't fight over family possessions. Certainly the only known ones in my family.

For the first move, my mother and I took a week of ten-hour days to sort and catalog and give to each family member, from the oldest son-in-law to the newest great-granddaughter, specific treasured mementos of my mother's life. Perhaps one sister would have preferred the antique desk instead of the antique buffet, or Great-grandmother's plates instead of the wicker porch chairs. No matter. Nary a cross word was spoken. I thought it was remarkable.

Each time my mother declined in health, in an ever-decreasing spiral of movement, my second sister and I moved her again. By the last move, we had had it. We had already given to Goodwill and the women's shelter and the community church. We had given and given and given away, but still my mother's possessions collected. Whether family treasures or dusty silk flower arrangements, we kept finding more with every box we moved to a new place.

"You take this!"

"No, you take it."

"I don't want it. I've got too much stuff already."

"Well, I don't have room."

"Who can we give it to?"

"Maybe this grandchild would like the couch."

"Maybe this granddaughter will take these lamps."

"You've got to store all the rest. Mother still wants these things, just in case."

"Just in case?"

"She thinks she may get better, and that someday she may want all these things."

"Oh, no! Just take this."

"I'm already storing stuff from the last move. You take it."

"No, you take it!"

We rocked in laughter and fatigue as we tried to give away my mother's possessions.

At the end of one sweltering day, carrying to my car armfuls of clothes we doubted my mother would ever wear again, my sister deftly thrust two hanging flower baskets into the backseat. They had graced either side of my mother's doorway for years, at the home she loved so much, whose front door had hand-painted ducks on it that said "Welcome."

I am not good with plants or flowers. I have the best intentions, but I forget to water them. I don't even talk to them.

After registering my protest to my sister, I took the flowers home. I set the hanging baskets in an untidy heap on my terrace, on a white, wrought-iron table that I had inherited from an earlier move of my mother's, and promptly forgot about them.

The summer lengthened and drooped with drought and heat. Everything living just about died. At ten o'clock each night, it was still in the high nineties. Too hot to walk. Too hot to do anything except sit on the terrace and watch the stars.

One night my gaze fell on a corner of the terrace. Flowers were growing there. Pink and purple blooms were pushing up from between the flagstones of the terrace. Yards away from these unexpected blooms, the hanging baskets sat, their flowers dried, dusty, dead. I don't know how the flowers had gotten into the terrace, but there they stayed. All summer long they bloomed. In direct sunlight, with no water. Even the lawn care man couldn't uproot them, the time or two he tackled the weeds around the terrace steps. Maybe the squirrels, who had eaten my other plants, had scattered the seeds. Or maybe it was the wind. It hardly matters.

I walk through my spacious house, more crowded now than I would ever choose, crowded with the cherished, much-used possessions of the generations of women I spring from. I give away a table, a set of glasses, some sheets and towels. I give away pictures. I give away clothes. I give away piles of books.

My mother is very ill. This has been the truth of her situation for four years. I pick up a needlepoint pillow she made for me. I hug it to my chest. I sleep in my grandmother's brass bed, the one her grandmother brought from Tennessee to Texas in a covered wagon. I read in bed by the light of the floor lamp that I read from as a child. I sleep under the crocheted afghan that once graced my mother's bed.

My mother's flowers bloom on.

Resident Bill of Rights

This notice hangs on the walls of various personal care, as-sisted-care, and nursing home facilities.

(1) Each personal care facility shall post the Resident's Bill of Rights, as provided by the Department, in a prominent place in the facility and be written in the primary language of each resident.

(2) In addition to other rights a resident has as a citizen, a resident has the rights provided by this section.

(3) The Resident's Bill of Rights must provide that each resident in the personal care facility has the right to:

(A) Not be physically or mentally abused or exploited;

(B) Not be physically or chemically restrained unless the restraint:

(i) Is necessary in an emergency to protect the resident or others from injury after the individual harms or threatens to harm himself or another; or

(ii) Is authorized in writing by a physician for a limited and specified period of time.

(C) If mentally retarded, participate in a behavior modification program involving use of restraints or adverse stimuli only with the informed consent of a guardian;

(D) Be treated with respect, consideration, and recognition of his or her dignity and individuality. A resident shall receive personal care

continued

and private treatment in a safe and decent living environment;

(E) Not be denied appropriate care on the basis of his or her race, religious practice, color, national origin, sex, age, handicap, marital status, or source of payment;

(F) Not be prohibited from communicating in his or her native language with other individuals or employees for the purpose of acquiring or providing any type of treatment, care, or services;

(G) Be encouraged and assisted in the exercise of his or her rights. A resident may present grievances on behalf of the resident or others to the manager, state agencies, or other persons without threat of reprisal in any manner. The person providing services shall develop procedures for submitting complaints and recommendations by residents and for assuring a response by the person providing the services;

(H) Receive and send unopened mail;

(I) Unrestricted communication, including personal visitation with any person of the resident's choice, including family members and representatives of advocacy groups and community service organizations, at any reasonable hour;

(J) Make contacts with the community and to achieve the highest level of independence, autonomy, and interaction with the community of which the resident is capable;

(K) Manage his or her financial affairs, or resident shall be given at least a quarterly ac-

continued

counting of financial transactions made on his or her behalf by the facility should the facility accept his or her written delegation of this responsibility to the facility for any period of time in conformance with state law;

(L) Have confidential records which cannot be released without his or her written permission. A resident may inspect his or her personal records maintained by the person providing services;

(M) Have the person providing services answer questions concerning the resident's health, treatment, and condition unless a physician determines that the knowledge would harm the resident. The physician must record the determination in the resident's record;

(N) Choose a personal physician;

(O) Participate in planning his or her service plan and medical treatment;

(P) Be given the opportunity to refuse treatment after the possible consequences of refusing treatment are fully explained;

(Q) Unaccompanied access to a telephone at a reasonable hour or in case of an emergency or personal crisis;

(R) Privacy;

(S) Retain personal clothing and possessions as space permits. The number of personal possessions may be limited for health and safety reasons which are documented in the resident's medical record. The number of personal possessions may be limited for the health and safety of other residents;

continued

(T) Determine his or her dress, hair style, or other personal effects according to individual preference, except the resident has the responsibility to maintain personal hygiene;

(U) Retain and use personal property in his or her immediate living quarters and to have an individual locked area (cabinet, closet, drawer, footlocker, etc.) in which to keep personal property;

(V) Refuse to perform services for the facility, except as contracted for by the resident and operator;

(W) Be informed, in writing, by the person providing services of available services and the applicable charges if the services are not covered by Medicare, Medicaid, or other form of health insurance;

(X) Not be transferred or discharged unless:

    (i) The resident's medical needs require transfer;

    (ii) The resident's health and safety or the health and safety of another resident requires transfer or discharge;

    (iii) The resident fails to pay for services, except as prohibited by federal law; or

    (iv) The resident repeatedly abuses alcohol, drugs, facility smoking regulations, or manifests severe and intentional antisocial behavior.

(Y) Not be transferred or discharged, except in an emergency situation. The responsible party of the resident and the attending physician shall be notified immediately;

continued

(Z) Leave the facility temporarily or permanently, subject to contractual or financial obligations; and

(AA) Not be deprived of any constitutional, civil, or legal right solely by reason of residence in a personal care facility;

(BB) Have access to the service of a representative of the state Long-term Care Ombudsman Program, Texas Department on Aging.

Section 146.125. Resident's Rights, Effective August 31, 1993. From Texas Department of Health Services.

Ending the Caregiving

We have to accept death; it makes life possible. The cells in our body are dying every day, but we never think to organize funerals for them. The death of one cell allows for the birth of another. Life and death are two aspects of the same reality.

—THICH NHAT HANH

A Minister Looks at Death

BY REVEREND MARGIE ANN NICOLA, D.D.

Death is a mystery to most people. Until we confront it in our immediate family, it's something we read about in the papers, it's something that happens to other people. We can feel great compassion and sympathy for others who are experiencing it and at the same time have no concept of what "it" is. Although one day it happens to everyone, most of us feel it is so far down the road in life that we submerge any thought of it. Because we refuse to believe that death occurs to both the young and the old, the well and the sick, the rich and the poor, we are un-educated and unprepared when our first confrontation with physical mortality occurs. That certainly was my experience.

My father was killed in an automobile accident when I was fifteen years old. Living in the Midwest, my mother and I followed the traditional funeral arrangements. For three days we sat from early morning until late night in the funeral home "receiving visitors." It was a dance that had to be danced no matter what the price. We were so caught up in other people's reactions that our own feel-ings were put aside. We simply existed in a vacuum, maintaining the semblance of what was expected. My mother was placed in the care of a doctor, whose answer for her pain was sleeping pills. When we would finally go home at night, she would fall into bed and I was left to survive as best I could. Somehow I was lost in the shuf-fle, which was no one's fault, just the way it was. Under-standable but regrettable.

I can remember standing at the screen door of the funeral home the second evening, looking out and wondering what I was supposed to do. I didn't know what a person did when she "grieved" for her father. I didn't particularly feel anything except isolation, confusion, and fear. This thing that lay in the casket wasn't my father. My dad was a volatile personality that was either laughing, angry, or intensely involved in something. I had been told he had been badly mangled in the accident, and yet the face and body showed no signs of injury. Maybe they were wrong. Maybe my dad wasn't dead, whatever that was.

The nightmare of the wake finally came to an end, the people went home and back to their lives, and Mother and I returned to an empty house, an empty life. I remember some friends of mine came by the house and asked if I wanted to go for a Coke, and I didn't know whether to go or not. Should I leave my mother? Was it proper? Was I supposed to look sad? I still felt numb.

Because there was no one to guide me through my grief, I stayed in the "loss" mode for years and years. My behavior patterns were affected and I formed belief systems based on the fear of something I didn't understand. The fear of rejection and abandonment was paramount in all of my relationships. I very effectively became a rejecter because I knew how to deal with that mode of action, whereas I still didn't understand, or know how to cope with, rejection and loss.

I am convinced that because death and dying were unknown and feared subjects, and because I was not encouraged to embrace and explore this unknown, I lived my life in fear of anything that was unknown.

In the ministry, one of the most challenging services I had to learn was ministering to the dying and to the family unit "left behind." My observations have reinforced my earlier experience. People simply are not prepared for death. Not the person making the transition nor the family group. Dying, death, and grieving are experiences that should not be shunted under the table, nor should it be taken for granted that everyone knows how to die and to grieve. Both are shrouded in mystery and certainly not something discussed in our culture. Perhaps this book will begin to change that.

It has been my observation that most of those who are dying desperately need someone who isn't afraid of them and their situation. Many times they need to talk about their condition and their impending death. Unfortunately, sometimes the family and friends simply cannot fill this need. Perhaps they are in denial and will not face the process. Perhaps it reminds them of their own mortality. Perhaps it represents too much of a loss for them to acknowledge.

As a counselor, much of my service is simply listening and loving. When people ask for advice, I encourage them to consider alternative ways of thinking and feeling. I remind them consistently that they are loved, that they are important, and that God loves them, because often the dying feel as though they are being punished by God for some known or unknown deed or thought.

When the illness is a long and slow deterioration, some come to a space and time when they make their peace with the process, life, and their God. Usually when peace is experienced, death follows soon. Others put up a valiant struggle to the last breath. Others seem to be waiting for permission from the family.

Those that are diagnosed as "terminally ill" are sometimes left to face their death alone. Many times the family and friends will fall by the wayside as the condition worsens and the time drags on, leaving the patient with a sense of alienation and isolation to struggle alone with death and pain. It seems to me that the family and friends cannot deal with their loved one's drama, for it becomes their drama. They simply cannot handle the emotions involved and so they avoid the whole situation. Understandable but regrettable.

Fortunately, I have aligned with a philosophy and belief system that has taught me life and death are one and the same and God is equally invested in both. As I have made my peace with my reality I can now allow my loved ones to make their choices, to live their lives as they need to and then to leave this plane of existence and enter another. I can afford to let them go, even though I experience "loss" and grieve for my loss, knowing that I will pass through the pain. Because of my spiritual life I know that my loved ones are loved and received in love as they experience all dimensions of life.

Death is not an ending, it is a beginning—for the deceased and for the survivor. Death is but the closing of one door and the opening of another in the adventure of living. The pain that is experienced is the result of clinging to one form of expression while entering another. For the deceased and the survivor, the pain is part of resisting change. I have seen lovers reunited at the last breath, I have seen spiritual understanding expand at the last breath, I have seen broken families restored, I have seen such great beauty and infinite peace expressed with the last breath.

I do not believe it is our fear of death that is the great challenge to us, but our fear of life. If we each understood the secrets of life we would not fear death.

Saying Good-bye to Someone You Love

Thanks to Chelsea Psychotherapy Associates, NYC, for
permission to reprint this excerpt from "Saying Good-bye to
Someone You Love," written by Dixie Beckham, Diego Lopez,
Luis Palacios-Jiminez, Vincent Patti and Michael Shernoff.

Death is a normal and inevitable part of everyone's life. Yet
few of us are prepared to deal effectively with someone
who is dying. Very often we are left feeling powerless and
helpless, that there is little we can do to make a difference
during this time.

Everyone dies differently and as they need to. Some people die fighting, others have given up, and still others may
die pretending they are not dying. Allow your loved ones to
face their final moments as they wish. Remember, there is
no right or wrong way to die. Denying one's own death is
common. If it doesn't hurt anyone, don't try to take this away
from the dying. After all, what have you got to replace the
denial with? Many people die in character, often exactly how
they lived. Not everyone can meet death in a noble or heroic
way. There is integrity in dying in one's own way.

Understand that your loved one may fear dying or even
welcome it. Dying can be very different from our expectations. Don't mold the reality of the moment into a roman-
tic idea of what it should be. Despite how difficult it is for
you, be there and remain real.

Dying people still have hope—of not suffering anymore,
of being remembered, of an afterlife. Try to support their
hope. They may not have anything else at this time.

Someone who is dying may be very angry and striking
out inappropriately at those who are closest to him or her.
Try not to take this personally.

Though a normal part of life, death can sometimes look, sound, and smell ugly. Prepare yourself and move on. Try not to let this interfere with the relationship you have with the person who is dying. Don't let the pain or unpleasantness get in the way of your love and being there.

LOGISTICS

The dying have special needs. Sometimes they need to plan their own funerals or make other arrangements. Inquire about whether you could be helpful in carrying out these last wishes.

Sometimes a dying person needs to give away things that she has cherished in the hope of helping keep her memory alive.

RECONCILIATION

What can you do for someone during his last weeks or days, his final moments? Tell him what he means to you, what you've learned from him. Tell him what will make you think about him. Reminisce about the wonderful, funny, or difficult times you shared. Touch and hold him. Understand that all we have between people are moments—of loving, of sharing, of being close and understood.

The end of life is a time for reconciliation and closure, for completing unfinished business. Spend time with your friend, whether crying, laughing, or silently holding hands. These experiences will provide profound and fresh memories.

It's not unusual to become aware of one's own mortality when someone we love is dying. Death destroys the illusion that we have enough time. Use what time you have left together to affirm you both, to say anything you may or may not have expressed yet.

Our illness or someone else's can make us question the nature of life. We may become angry at God. It's okay. Remember, God is big enough to survive our anger.

Take stock of spiritual beliefs and reaffirm them. God or whatever deity you may believe in can be a source of comfort, healing, and tranquility.

GRIEF

Death is the final part of living. It may be the ultimate life crisis, requiring special coping and adjusting. Just how do we say good-bye to a life of sharing and loving? Although our loved one is physically gone, our feelings don't go with him or her. This is the nature of grief.

The mourning process often begins at the time of diagnosis and continues long after the person has died.

It is often common for the surviving caregiver to feel relief immediately following the death of a loved one. This is especially likely to be true if the dying process has been drawn out and difficult.

You may not believe death has really happened. Some people experience disbelief and shock.

The absence of grief immediately following the death of a loved one may be a warning sign that you may have a lot of difficulty later on. This may be a form of denial. While we all use denial and it is normal and often useful, we must remember that the pain is still there, even if we're not feeling it.

You may notice others acting inappropriately. Allow them to express their grief in their own way.

Grief is a process of healing that takes time. Learn to nurture yourself. Don't allow the intensity of the pain to frighten you.

The hurt can feel like a bottomless pit, but you do eventually feel better. To hurt from a loss is okay and normal.

You may feel that life isn't worth living without the deceased. This is only a passing feeling, not an answer.

Intense weeping is one of the main expressions of grief. It is often a necessary release of feelings as well as a means of establishing contact with others during these painful moments. Crying can be healthy and cleansing. But not everyone is a crier, so don't try to force this if it is not a natural way for you to react.

While grieving, certain things may occur: shortness of breath, tightness in your throat, frequent sighing, sadness, fatigue, difficulty concentrating, loss of appetite, difficulty sleeping, loss of sex drive, a belief that you're hearing the voice of the deceased.

During this time it's not uncommon for some people to yearn to be reunited with their loved one. You may search for her in a crowded room or on the street; you may expect him to be home waiting for you, or you may call his name at night. You may actually imagine seeing her in places she used to frequent.

If you experience any of the things described in the above two paragraphs, don't become alarmed. Many people report that some of these things have happened to them following the death of someone they loved.

The traditional rituals of mourning, such as wakes, funerals, burials, shiva, memorial services, cemetery stones, or novenas, can serve an important function in bringing closure. The ceremonies help make accepting the reality of death easier and provide a structure and form to the grieving process. Don't deprive yourself of them if they are meaningful to you.

Mourning is a way of saying good-bye. Don't avoid it. You need time for healing. Pictures, letters, and other pieces of the deceased's personal property can be helpful during this process. Use them to help get you through this period.

Try to take better care of yourself now more than ever.

After someone's death it's not uncommon to need a vacation, to get away or lie on a beach. Getting some space and distance can be immensely helpful and healing.

Rest and take care of yourself, but beware of isolating yourself from friends, family, and the living. Throughout it all, remember that others can help. This is not a time to feel alone. A friend, family member, social worker, or clergy person may be useful to reach out to. Mourning needs resolution in order for you to go on with your life.

The period of mourning immediately following a death is not the time to make any major decisions. Wait. If it is the correct thing to do, time will tell.

You may be very angry without realizing it. Try not to turn the anger or rage against yourself. Let it out. It's okay. A truly horrible thing has just happened to you. The loss of a spouse, parent, child, or close friend is an excellent reason to be angry.

You may be very angry at the deceased for dying. This is normal. Forgiveness plays an important part in grief. You may need to forgive him or her for dying and leaving you. You may need to forgive yourself for all the things you could have done or would have done differently.

Grieving is a process of letting go of what might have been or should have been. It is a time for making peace with the reality of your loss and for saying good-bye.

A loved one's death can trigger old memories of other losses—a mother, a brother, a divorce, being fired. These memories may make this time even more painful.

Realize you may also be mourning the dreams you had for the deceased. As a spouse, it may be the house you wanted to buy or that special trip you never got to take. As a parent, it may be the hopes you had for your child. It is especially difficult for a parent to have a child die. It is not part of the natural order of things for a parent to bury his or her child.

Birthdays, anniversaries, and holidays following the death of a loved one may be especially painful.

We don't always have control over memories. That special song can reawaken old feelings. Just acknowledge to yourself that, although painful, this is another normal aspect of grief. Feelings remind us that we are still alive, as well as rekindling memories of our dead loved one.

After the initial shock and disbelief, a period of disorganization may happen. The hardest time of all may be long after everyone else is gone. Things are settled down and life returns to what it was before, only your loved one has died. Be aware that the loss is settling in. You may feel empty inside.

You cannot continue to live your life as if the deceased were still alive. This does not mean that you have to give up your loved one. The task is to find ways to let that person live on in your memory.

Try not to worry, "Am I grieving correctly?" You'll do it in your own style and at your own pace. There is not one correct way to grieve.

Don't deny your urges to exercise your faith, religion, or spirituality. It may provide some needed answers.

A point of understanding and acceptance eventually occurs. The preoccupation with what has happened and with your dead loved one does diminish over time. The intense feelings lessen, and memories become less painful. A renewed interest in other people and life in general does occur.

It's okay to survive the death of someone you love.

The Dying Person's Bill of Rights

BY E. M. BAULCH

The right to be treated as a living human being until death.

The right to have a sense of hopefulness, however changing its focus may be.

The right to be cared for by those who can maintain a sense of hopefulness, however changing this may be.

The right to express feelings and emotions about one's own approaching death in one's own way.

The right to participate in decisions concerning one's own care.

The right to expect continuing medical and nursing care even though the "cure" goals may be changed to "comfort" goals.

The right not to die alone.

The right to be free of pain.

The right to have questions answered fully and honestly.

The right to retain one's own individuality and not be judged for decisions that may be contrary to others' beliefs.

The right to be cared for by caring, sensitive, knowledgeable people who will attempt to understand one's needs.

The right to die in peace and dignity.

The right to expect that the sanctity of the human body will be respected after death.

Lessons Learned from the Dying:
A Conversation with Caregivers

"Death is a great adventure. I can hardly wait."

> —JOEY S., an 83-year-old
> man with cancer, five
> days before he died

Laurie W., a home health care nurse who works with terminally ill patients, took care of David K.'s father, Joey S., for the last few weeks of his life. I interviewed Joey, Laurie, and David a few days before Joey died.

David is one of the most loving young men I have ever met. A male nurse who saw a need and opened himself up to fill that need, he started the first home health care agency for AIDS patients in Los Angeles County.

As Laurie and David and I talked, I became aware of what a remarkable opportunity it was to hear their deepest feelings about the whole range of caregiver issues. Their insights helped me, as I know they will help you, to understand the caregivers who work with the dying—their grief, their burnout, their coping strategies. We talked also about our ideal visions for the future for caregivers and for the dying. I had just interviewed David's father, who was now sleeping peacefully. He was an inspiring example to all of us of a vital, unique man dying at peace with himself.

BCM: Laurie, I'd like to know how this tour of duty differs from other people that you have taken care of who have gone through the dying process.

LW: Well, this job is a pleasure for me because Joey's eighty-three years old, it's natural. It appears as though he's very accepting of death and that he's ready to go. I should note that I usually take care of AIDS patients that are young men; it's not time for them. They fight and they struggle as you try to help them through the process of dying. It's devastating because you don't know what to do, you don't know how to help them get through it so that they can start coming to terms with dying, and help the people they love that are there, help them get through it, too.

BCM: Yes, I seems like such a tragedy when it's a young person.

LW: It's terrible. It's terrible.

BCM: And when it's an older person, it's like this beautiful gentleman says, it's the next step.

LW: It is, it's the natural turn of events. We know when we're born we are destined to die. But you're not destined to die at twenty-five, twenty-six, twenty-seven, twenty-eight.

BCM: There's such a sense of unfinished business. Almost a sense of being robbed of your life.

LW: They are robbed. And they suffer terribly. I've noticed with AIDS patients that there is such a high level of stress that they can't sleep, they're afraid to sleep, they're afraid not to sleep, there's a lot of disorientation. And I don't know how to help. I don't know how to get to them so that I can put them at peace. So that they can rest. So that they can come to terms with dying. Because they're in such denial, they're not open to what you have to say when you try to tell them that if they rest things will be better in the morning, that their minds are just kind of stretched out and tired. I've really noticed that in them. Just a constant exhaustion. They fight. They struggle.

BCM: Yes. Bill, another nurse who deals with AIDS patients, told me that his first case was a young man, and he kept trying to make him comfortable, but the patient sat on the edge of the bed all night long, because he was so afraid that if he went to sleep he would die. The stress they both went through! Then of course, with Michael, my son who died of AIDS, what we went through was the most transfiguring experience and at the same time it was the most devastating experience, week after week and month after month, year after year, to move from emotion to emotion, from experience to experience.

LW: And to watch them waste away.

BCM: Yes, and to move from the struggle to the acceptance. I wondered if the nurses go through all of that range of emotions—the rage and the terror and the guilt and the grief.

LW: I seem to attach to my patients very quickly. Because I have children.

BCM: So do I, I say, "Thank you, God" every day for all of my children still living.

LW: Oh, that's what I say. "Thank you, God, that my child doesn't have AIDS." So when I go in there I have a pretty motherly attitude toward them, because I think, "Gee, this could be my kid." And so I strive when I take care of them to treat them the way I would want my son treated. I respect everything that they are going through. Anything they want I do it, whatever they want. So I do go through a lot of things with them because I just attach. And when they die I have a real hard time of it. I don't want to go through it again for a while. I just had a patient who died recently. Then I came on this case and I said, "Oh, thank God," because I don't feel the same when I'm here with Joey as I do when I'm taking care of the young ones. I mean, I don't feel uncomfortable here with him dying. It feels just right. He's made it right.

BCM: But when you have patient after patient, the young ones that you've had that are dying of AIDS or other terminal diseases, what do you do afterwards to get yourself to the point where you can go into the next situation again and take care of someone who is terminally ill?

LW: Well, immediately I go home and cry, and fortunately for me, I've only had two patients die while I've been there. When they die and you're not there it's not as bad as when they die and you are there, because you're more separated from the situation. So both of the times that I've had a patient die, I've gone home and I've been fortunate because my boyfriend is there, so I just collapse in his arms and he just hugs me and pampers me and babies me and then I mourn.

After this last one died, I just said, "Okay, today is a day of mourning." And that's what we do at the house. Everybody pampers me and babies me and it's a day of mourning.

BCM: Doesn't it take longer than a day, though?

LW: Yes, it does. And then what I do is I don't work with dying patients for a while. I go back into the hospital. I work in the hospital, which is not the greatest environment, but at least it's not all death and dying, it's people that are going to get better, people that are going to go home. There's hope. So I do that. Yes, it does take a long time to grieve. And this last one, this young man who died, when I think about him I am still in mourning.

BCM: Have your ideas on dying and on nursing, on taking care of terminally ill patients, changed over the years with these experiences?

LW: My ideas on death and dying have changed considerably. I was talking to David last night about how death puts you more in touch with your own mortality. Yes, you are going to die and everyone is going to die. I think it's given me a healthier approach to life and to death. I think that since I have gone through this a few times and seen these patients die, it's really made me a better nurse. It gives me more insight into other people's lives. It makes me a more caring person. I think that contact with death and dying has done a lot for me.

BCM: You talked about how your views had changed on death and dying. Do you fear death?

LW: Not as much as I used to, which is interesting. You know, you'd think that after being around it for a while you'd fear it a little bit more. But no, I don't. I fear it less than I did before. You know, after they die, they're so peaceful. Aren't they? They are so peaceful. And it's just like something has happened that has made them that peaceful, that the struggle is finally over. Even the worst strugglers are peaceful.

BCM: What about your own struggle with life? Are you less of a struggler now that you have been with patients who have died?

LW: Am I struggling with life itself or denying death? I probably do struggle less than I did. When these things happen, I feel like I need to find something in every day of my life to enjoy and I need to bring myself more pleasure, that I need to do more things for myself. That's another thing I'm getting out of it. I went into nursing because I am a caregiver, but I found out that I need to get something back. So I'm more demanding. I notice that in my own house I'm now demanding that my family give me more. I've always done everything in the house. You know, I go out and work twelve hours and I go home and it's still okay for me to cook and clean and do all the stuff that I've always done when I didn't work twelve hours. Well, I've found out now that people need to give back to me what I give to them. I deserve it. My kids have started doing things to help me.

BCM: So it's more of a balance. You have to fill up so that you will have something to give the next time.

LW: It is more of a balance. And they've started doing more. Not that they do the laundry, but I've gotten them to pick up the laundry, to put the laundry in its proper place, which is a big thing. It's really interesting how everybody has kind of pitched in.

DK: And you know, one thing that Laurie said earlier that makes her case very fortunate is that so many times nurses experience this type of grief and then go home to their family and friends, where they're met with, "Well, you're a nurse, don't you know how to deal with death? I mean, isn't death a part of your work? What's the big deal?" Or, "Oh, I thought you were supposed to maintain a professional distance. Aren't you goofing up here?"

BCM: These are important issues that you mention, David, and I do want to elicit specifically the things you do for your own mourning process, your own recovery process. And that could be both the practical and the esoteric ways that you deal with all this. Being in the world in a certain very special way, dealing with death and dying, and then going back to people who just don't know.

LW: I think that one of the things that happens as part of the dying process is that people feed off of you and you feed off of them. You gain strength from them and they gain strength from you. They give you the courage to go on. There was so much appreciation from my last patient, from his friend, and from his family. His mother and father came, and they gave me so much back. So sometimes it seems like you're not giving as much as you're getting back. I even feel like that here. I feel like I'm getting a lot from Joey. I don't know how much he's getting from me and I do make him happy, but . . .

DK: Don't sell yourself short. He loves you.

LW: I know he does, David. And I love him. I do get so much from all of them. Then when they die, and you leave when they die, well, you know how it feels when somebody dies. You feel terrible. You go into mourning and that's another thing. People don't know how to mourn. No one has ever been taught how to mourn. It's a very personal, very private thing.

BCM: You can't do it wrong.

LW: You can't do it wrong. Thank God.

DK: Paradise into reality is people who mourn well.

BCM: Yes. One week after my son died, the tears were coming, I couldn't hold them back, and people would say, "What's the matter with you? Don't you know he's happy and at peace? Get on with your life." One week! And my rage would come up. How dare they negate these feelings I'm going through?

LW: But I think there's another thing that happens some-times when a loved one dies. You have this other reac-tion where you may say to yourself, "Oh my God, it's only a week and I'm stopping mourning. This can't be right." But yet, the person who has died doesn't want you to mourn. And they'll tell you that.

BCM: It is *your* recovery process.

LW: Here is a person who has fought and struggled till the last breath has been drawn, to live, and when we go into such terrible mourning, we're not living. We're not doing what they wanted us to do.

BCM: The loss is for us. It's not a loss for them. When Michael died, I called my mother and she said, "Thank God, he's at peace." In the midst of our sorrow we were rejoicing because we loved him so much and we didn't want to see him suffer in that deteriorating body week after week. But oh, the mourning! At first there was peace and relief. But then, when you realize that the person you love is gone, this magnificent young person. . . . You need to take a very long time to go through healing the part of you that has experienced that devastating loss because it is such a loss.

LW: It's worse for a family member. As a mother, it's so sad. I had a baby that died at birth, so I know what it feels like to lose somebody you love. Some people say, "Well, you never knew the baby." And that's just not true, that's not the way it is.

BCM: It's a part of you.

LW: It is. And you suffer. It's an unnatural turn of events to have your children die before you. It's more natural for your father to die, David. That is a natural turn of events, especially at your age and at his age. But not for you to die. If the positions were reversed, if it was you in that bed and your father was taking care of you, I don't think we would be having these conversations. Because there would be so much pain.

I'm just saying from personal experience, no matter how "spiritually aware" you believe you are, there is such rage at your child being taken from you. Someone that is a part of you being ripped up like a tree, a young tree. I think that colors a lot of what is going on. That you're helpless to protect your child.

BCM: Oh yes! But David and I were talking about how when his father goes, it's the last person in the world left ahead of him in his life. You're all alone and you're a grown-up now, David. In fact, there's nobody between you and death or between you and the rest of the world.

DK: Yes, and somehow there's an inner peace that it is supposed to be that way. In fact, I think that in a way, we prepare for this moment ahead of time.

Let me give you some background on my father's situation. I remember when my father called me and he told me about this dream he had. It all started when he had this dream. Earlier in this year he was walking two miles a day, he would do shows, he loved to go to Vegas with his friends and have a good time, he was a man in love with life. But then he called me up in December and he said, "I have to see you right away, son." I said, "What's wrong?" And he said, "Well, let me just come down to L.A. and I'll tell you." I said, "Sure, but I'm worried. What's wrong?" And he said, "Well, I dreamed last night that I was about to die. I saw it all and it was all real clear and I feel like it's really true. I don't want this to be a tragedy. I feel it's my time and I just want to come down and see you and let's play."

So I agreed. He flew here and after about four days here we went to Vegas and spent five days there together and just had a great time together. And we talked about it all, the dream, his conviction that it was his time to die. I thought, Well, who knows if it's real or not, but you never know; and it's just amazing that it turns out now to be true. He is going to die. Yet both he and I are at peace about it.

LW: I wish each dying could be as peaceful. For that is the order of the universe. We do think that some day we will lose our parents. We don't think, "Someday I'll be burying my children."

BCM: No, we don't.

DK: The other thing about mourning is that I believe that mourning is something that should be shared. Share that point in yourself that's grieving. It's so wonderful to be able to do that because you know that there will be a time that allows the mourning process to subside. There will be a part of your heart that will mourn forever and yet you will not grieve forever.

BCM: I think it's wonderful that we are sharing this now with each other because death itself has been such a taboo subject in the Western world. It's amazing to me that caregivers beginning in this type of work can move through their own conscious and unconscious fears of death. To me, that seems to be the great lesson and I wondered if you would like to comment on that.

LW: Well, I wanted to say something about the way I feel about the mourning process with regard to mourning people who are relative strangers—although they aren't by the time they die, even if it's only a couple of weeks that you're taking care of them. You know everything about them by that time. But it's not as bad as a real close friend or a family member or a lover dying. Because then you really know them, and you've experienced life's joys with them and you're going to miss them. Whereas as a nurse you haven't experienced life's joys with them, you've only experienced life's trials and pain with them.

BCM: That's a really good insight. I hadn't thought of that before.

LW: You usually haven't seen joy in those people. You've just seen them miserable. Although, through this old guy out here, I experience some of life's joys with him.

BCM: As I was coming over here a part of me was thinking, "This is the most wonderful opportunity to meet with David's father and to share with both of them," and another part of me was really dreading this today. I thought, "Oh, we're going to bring back all of my grief for Michael." And instead I feel so invigorated because of the joy that is in the room!

LW: That is the way I feel. When I come here I feel good about being here.

DK: Oh, I feel good about you being here too!

LW: Whether he's dying or not dying.

DK: Well, isn't that the key for us, to feel good whether or not he's dying?

LW: Yes.

DK: Let me just share with you the most amazing experience my father and I had when he was in the intensive care ward. It changed how I feel about death in a profound and personal way.

It was after his heart attack. One night we were talking in the intensive care unit and we were laughing some and crying some. Then he went to sleep and the doctor came in and told me the news that my father had cancer, as well as the problems with his heart. They did not think, at that time, that he would live through the night.

My father was sleeping and I was crying. He woke up and he asked me, "What's going on? Why are you crying?" So I pulled myself together somewhat and I told him the truth about what the doctors and nurses had said. "Well your heart's not doing well tonight. And they don't think you're going to make it through the night."

He just lay there and looked at me for a minute or two and then he said, "Well, I don't know what to say. I've had a good life, and I've had eighty-three years, and you know you talk all the time about people with AIDS, the ones you work with in your service. They're dying at twenty-five. I have nothing to complain about."

Isn't that a remarkable statement from a dying man? "I have nothing to complain about."

BCM: Yes, it is.

DK: Then we talked a little bit more and he said, "Well, son, I know that this is going to be hard on you, but time heals." Then he said, "In a lot of ways in the past few years my life has been boring. I wake up every morning with the mind of a forty-year-old, and then I'm reminded that I'm an eighty-three-year-old man. I can't do the things I want to do. I can't be the person that I want to be anymore. It just feels right that it's time to move on." Then we were both quiet for a while. And finally he said to me, "In a lot of ways I'm real excited about it."

So we started laughing and crying and reminiscing together and even speculating a little on what it would be like on the other side. We started exploring. We talked about death and the hereafter. We were saying to each other, "Well, what do you think it's going to be like with each of us? Do you think that all of a sudden you'll be there on the other side and there will be Mom greeting you there, and your parents and your brother? Or you'll just be this spirit or this light and there will be another spirit or another light next to you, and you'll realize that this is the same feeling that you got from my mother and you'll realize that it's her? Or you'll be surrounded by a warmth all of a sudden and you'll realize that you haven't felt that particular warmth since your parents were here? On this side? And now they are there, with you, on the other side? What's it going to be like?"

And then we talked about reincarnation too. "What if you're going to wake up in this brand-new body raring to go? How exciting that will be!" Then he could start over. We talked about all the old sayings, you know, like "youth is wasted on the young," and what if he had a brand-new body but he had this great old wisdom, and "if I knew then what I know now"—all those things. And we thought, "What if you get to take all your experiences with you? What if you *do* get to wake up in a brand-new body with all this experience and get to be young again with all that you know? How incredible *that* would be! The possibilities are endless." We even wondered, "Do you think there will be cities where you are going? How familiar or unfamiliar will it be?" We wondered and played with the possibilities all night long.

BCM: How extraordinary!

DK: Right. And then, once we had gone through the painful part of it, the possibilities were endless. It became more of a celebration of what was happening to him than a death watch. When I thought of him going to this other place, maybe taking all his experiences or maybe having a whole new body, I thought, "It's really the miracle of death." You know, you hear so much about the miracle of birth that no one thinks what a miracle death must be.

That night in intensive care, it was almost like he made a miraculous recovery. It's almost like the more we accepted death, the more I embraced life. The more we don't run from death, the more we learn.

BCM: That's very profound, David.

DK: You mentioned the idea about death being a taboo. This is on the market now [*picks up a large book called* A Complete Guide for Patients and Their Families]. It's one of the books in home and health care. It has everything in it. Every type of patient, every illness. Just everything. Anything you want to know about home health care is in this book. If you look up in the index under "death," you know what you'll find?

BCM: What?

DK: Nothing! They didn't mention it.

BCM: You're kidding.

DK: This is our society.

BCM: David, what did you learn in school about death?

DK: Laurie and I went to school together actually. But we didn't learn anything about death in school. Nothing.

LW: Not one thing. I never remember anybody ever talking to us about death, David. It was just something that we did not talk about. You know when I started doing this, I thought, What do I do when somebody dies? How do I handle it? I just sort of went in and the first patient I had, he was forty, and it was a real comfortable situation for me because he was close to my age and I felt like I could sit and talk to him. Yet, when I first got to his house, I said to myself, "Oh my God, what am I going to do here? How am I going to handle all this?" Because I was so unprepared for it. All we had learned in school was that you're supposed to help people through the dying process.

BCM: How?

LW: How. Exactly. How do you do it? Well, in a way it wasn't so bad that they didn't try to teach us in school how to handle death and dying because, as a nurse, I do everything by rote. If I don't have it memorized then I don't know how to do it.

BCM: You've got to memorize death, is that it?

LW: Yes. So, remembering my first time, I went in this house and I thought, "Oh my God, what do I do?" It was my first day. And I think it's always the same the first day, things are a little tense, everybody is testing everybody else, you're not real comfortable, you want to do it right because everybody's there watching you and you think, "If I trip over this chair one more time they're going to throw me out of here because I'm a klutz." Well, as I was there longer and longer, this man and I developed a wonderful relationship. Then I thought, "This is what it is. This is why they didn't teach us this in school, because it's an experience." Everytime I go someplace now, I wait to see what the patient is going to do. And I follow their lead. I am just being myself, but I see what they want to talk about. In school they told us, "Get them in there to talk about death." Well they don't all want to talk about death. Sometimes they want to review their lives. Sometimes they don't want to review their lives.

BCM: Sometimes they just want to be taken care of.

LW: That's right. And some of them want to be children again. So that's what I do now. I just see what they want to do. What they want to talk about.

BCM: When I talk with caregivers I find that everyone I meet, well, you all have such a different attitude from the general attitude. It's almost like there's the civilians and then there are the people who are in the know about what is really going on.

DK: And the two shall never communicate.

BCM: It's as if people in our society think that dealing with dying is dangerous. As if it were contagious. They feel like if they don't think about it, it will go away. Yet I'm always so amazed at the beautiful life processes that I see happening when people do accept death.

DK: My life is more full and I'm more clear and more happy than I've ever been. I'm sure since I have such an issue with loss that it's no accident of the universe that I have a nursing service. But as much as there is loss, there's as much that I get. Sometimes when I do sit by these people's bedside, I am in awe and I think I'm the student, they are the teacher. Let me just hear what they have to say. The things you learn are incredible. And realistically, you know that the teachers and nurses could have never taught it to you.

LW: No, they could never have taught it. And it's always the same thing in nursing school. You would have had to memorize it, anyway. If you didn't do it right it was wrong.

BCM: Even though it is the most profound experience that you have ever gone through and the work that goes on is so intense, what do you do the rest of the time when you are not taking care of a patient? Laurie talked about mourning and of being taken care of by people in her family. Do you have anything else that you'd like to tell us?

DK: I think the most important thing is what she said. Realize that you are a human being and thank God human beings feel! You're entitled to have those feelings and to make time for them. The other thing I want to mention about seeing people dying time after time is that you live in constant crisis. The problem is so big that you can give twenty-four hours of yourself and you still won't make a dent in the AIDS crisis, or in any terminally ill situation. So the reality is that you have to know what you can give and see yourself in it for the long term and make sure that you give your twelve hours or so, and then take time off. Or take time after that death. Because if you don't you will burn out, and you will burn out fast.

LW: That's what I do. I take time off. When they called me the very same day that this last patient of mine died and they said, "We think we've got something for you," I just burst into tears on the telephone. I said, "Not now. I just can't take it."

BCM: Good for you. You've realized that you do get to the edge.

LW: Yes. I said, "Do you think I'm bionic or something? Get out of my life, I'm mourning."

DK: A lot of times a nurse will call the nursing service and say, "I can't do it anymore." So I'll call them and talk to them. It's amazing when you talk to people who are burning out. You can ask them, "What things did you enjoy one year ago?" And they'll say, "Well, I love plays, I love movies, I love dinner, I love going to the beach." Then you'll ask them, "In the past two months have you done those things?" They will say, "No." So the truth is, even if you know that everyone out there is dying and it's breaking your heart, you still need to take some time and have fun.

LW: I find I've been doing more of that, going for the joy, after taking care of these patients. Because I've got to live my life. It's what they want. That's what they've taught me. Get out there and do it! Live!

DK: We're caregivers and we give and give, not realizing that if we're not careful we can give it all away.

BCM: It's not that the giving ever stops but how can you give them an empty cup if you aren't filling up? I know mothers go through this, there's always a little, guilty voice saying, "You know, you may have just helped someone die, but you didn't do this, or you didn't do that." So how do you answer those little voices when you do take the time out to play, when you do take time out to take care of yourself?

LW: I never feel like that about the patients.

BCM: You never feel guilty about enjoying yourself even when someone you care about is dying?

LW: Right. Because they want you to enjoy yourself.

BCM: I needed to hear this. I want people to know the range of emotions that caregivers go through when they're dealing with this all the time.

DK: I've had two experiences recently of seeing so many people around me dying that after a while I felt horribly guilty about enjoying myself. But as Laurie said, you re-alize that those people you love want you to enjoy yourself. Also, I've sat with people when they are dying and it's amazing. It's like a microcosm of the universe; the time seems to stand still sometimes, and there is such a sense, when someone's dying, of how precious life is. And then you realize that you need to enjoy life to its fullest. Every day, every minute, every second.

Even with my father dying in there in the other room, what you're saying is true. Tonight I'm thinking of going out to dinner with friends. Well, I could sit here with him instead and ask myself, "Have I done enough?" Or if I go out, and he dies tonight, will I think, "God, last night I shouldn't have gone out to dinner to have a good time"?

BCM: The last night of Michael's life I went home to my son's house in a suburb of San Francisco to wash my hair. And I thought then, and sometimes even now I think . . .

DK: "What kind of mother is that!"

BCM: I know! I wanted to meditate on the balcony to let him go, because I felt like even though we had been in acceptance since Christmas, and this was now July, and we all kept praying that God would take him out of his pain and misery, I had the sense—and I'm wondering if you all have had this sometimes too—that many times a patient chooses to go only when he is alone because people are holding him or her back. They feel, "I don't want my mother to have to see this. I don't want to make it any harder on the people who are here." It's almost—especially since Michael was so considerate—as if he thought, "I will wait to die when they are not here to hold on to me in any way." Or maybe it's just a private thing.

DK: I'll tell you, it's often like that exactly. We've seen hundreds of patients at the nursing service, and the reality is, I have seen lovers and parents who have been obsessed with being there for that moment. I have seen people who have not left the house for two months. The groceries, et cetera, everyone else is handling it so that they can be there for that moment. I've seen it happen so many times, they'll be in the bathroom and then the dying one chooses to die alone no matter what. Either it is a private thing they want to go through or somehow internally they make a decision that it would be easier if Mother is not right there at the bedside, or anyone else.

BCM: And for some of them it's not that beautiful when they die. It's more like, "Do not go gentle into that good night. Rage, rage, against the dying of the light."

DK: We tell people that if it's meant to be, you will be there at the time of death. And it doesn't really matter that you spend twenty-four hours there, you just look for the quality in your time together. You look for what you do have together.

BCM: It's those issues of control. For both the dying and their loved ones.

DK: Right.

BCM: I saw this with Michael. He was determined to orchestrate his funeral, his celebration party afterward, every single aspect of his life. He was not going to give up control. That was his great lesson in life: to surrender, to let go of that control. A lot of times that's what the families are going through. They think death has to look a certain way, and it doesn't fit their pictures that they should be angry at this family member or that they should want to run wildly out of the house and take a two-hour walk, or that it is a very messy process sometimes, just like birth is.

DK: Exactly. I think we often protect people from the reality of death. I know that my father's death and my being here with him now looks textbook wonderful. And I want to tell you that my father and I have had lots of problems and lots of issues, and there has been lots of guilt there and lots of agony. When he was coming down here to spend time with me, I spent time with my therapist and I said, "You know I've been planning to have this talk with him and say to him, 'I love this and I appreciate this and I also want you to know that I'm real upset about this and I think that this was a horrible thing, and so on, but how can I say this to him now because death could be around the corner and, besides, he's eighty-three years old!" So my therapist and I talked about this, about how there's a difference between getting something out and getting even.

BCM: Very good point.

DK: It was important for me to get it out. Get it all out. Whatever I wanted or needed or desired to say to him. And it doesn't matter whether he may be dying or whether he's eighty-three. Once again you can't protect people from their own lives. The reality was, I felt so angry about some things, and he felt so guilty about other things during our whole relationship. So I sat down and I told him all the things that were upsetting to me, and he told me some things that I had done that were so upsetting to him. And as much as I thought that would be such a horrible confrontation, my anger was gone and his guilt was gone.

BCM: You cleared a space.

DK: We cleared everything. If you have something to say to someone, it doesn't matter if they're ninety-eight or if they're dying, say it!

BCM: It's always like that. And then you have such a sense of completeness, as you and I were talking about earlier.

So that's some valuable advice from someone who's been there.

DK: Right. Learn the difference between getting even and talking it out, and don't feel guilty about getting it all out.

BCM: What else?

LW: I think that there are some other things I have learned from death. You see, I was divorced when my kids were really young, and I did have some hard times with my children, what I called my little screamers with them, but we always talked. But now, taking care of dying patients, I've realized that I don't have to always be screaming inside, or screaming outside at other people either. So now instead of just yelling and freaking out because of something that my kids have done, I have the real ability to sit down and discuss things with them in a loving way. And that's what I think that death and dying has done for me.

BCM: You see that there's another way to do things.

LW: There is another way to do things. And everything can be done through love. You don't have to be destructive, you don't have to be hateful, you don't have to be anything, you just have to discuss things.

BCM: What do you do when you have very stubborn patients that you can't reach with love? I'm reminded of someone I know who got even by dying. How do you deal with dying when it doesn't look like a beautiful ending or everyone healing the relationship within? I still have trouble with this. Not every death is ideal.

DK: True! We were talking about this very thing this morning. When you go into someone's house and into someone's life, as much as you may think that emotionally you may have the answers for them, or you could help them communicate better, or you could facilitate a more beautiful death than the one they're having, you have to realize that they have had years to develop their relationships. The reality is that Nancy Nurse walking in twenty-four hours before someone's dying is not going to change this person's dynamics.

BCM: The families have to change it.

DK: Right. If a family lived in anger and lived in upset, that's probably just how the death is going to be. And that's acceptance of death. We can't only learn to accept beautiful death, we have to learn to accept any death, and people tend to die the same way they lived.

BCM: I have seen some remarkable changes occur in families when a death comes on the scene, and I'm also aware of what it involves, but it doesn't always work out the way that it's supposed to.

DK: Right. I remember one example from when I was working at a hospital on the geriatric cases. A skilled nursing facility was attached to the hospital, and an old man was there who was really angry and very, very mean. I kept wondering, "Have they mistreated him here, what happened here that has caused him to be so mean?" And his family came in one day and told me, "He's been mean all his life. This is him." We tend to think that what's going on now is what's determining the patient's emotions, yet people have had a lifetime to become who they are.

BCM: Yes. I tend to think everybody's so nice. I mean, isn't it that way? I tend to go around thinking everybody on the face of this earth is full of love when it simply isn't true.

DK: The reality of it all is that someone got even with this, and then they got even with that, and so they may then get even by dying. That's like suicide. Suicide can be . . .

LW: A real get-even.

DK: It can be one of the most selfish things that you can do to other human beings, or, I've seen it done in ways that it can be most beautiful. It can be someone taking control of his or her life by ending that life in a compassionate way.

BCM: The work I'm doing on death and dying and the grieving process has opened my eyes to the fact that there are just as many ways, and just as many reasons, for taking control of your life through the dying process as through the living process.

LW: I know. This last guy that I took care of had already made a pact with his loved one that if they both got sick they would just end their lives.

BCM: We were talking before about how your feelings have changed since you were in nursing school, yet it's been my understanding, and stop me if I'm wrong, that when you're a nurse or a doctor you pledge to save life no matter what. Keep people alive, no matter what they want. What is the reality? And how do your ideas change so that you know what is right about people living in such devastating ways, for example, hooked up to life support systems or in dementia or in great pain?

DK: The first thing I've learned is that there is no right and wrong. First thing. The second thing is to go for the quality, and not the quantity, of the person's life. Because we have so many tools now and so many machines that are incredible. We can prolong and sustain life, but at what cost? And I mean both the emotional and the financial cost.

LW: Ultimately, it's supporting the hospitals, it's supporting the doctors. They sometimes don't care about the patient, they sometimes don't have any real feelings about the patient, as you know. You have just gone through it.

Many doctors don't really care about the family members.

DK: Some of them don't.

LW: Why do they want to keep a person living?

DK: It is amazing to see the difference, though, in my father's case.

The first thing my father's doctor, an extremely overworked man, did with him was to sit down and say, "Joe, tell me about your life. What do you want? How do you see it? What do you think about death?" It wasn't like with most doctors who say, "Here's surgery, here's confinement, here's the plan." Instead he said to my father, "Joey, what's your plan?" It was incredible.

BCM: Do you see the future turning more toward recognizing the right of the person to die at home, toward home health care, and the softening of these impersonal, mechanistic attitudes? Like when the old family doctor used to be there for the person, and for the whole family?

LW: I guess we're turning to the old ways when people died at home with their family around and they were loved.

DK: We've totally avoided that in our culture. We've set up "funeral homes" because we don't want to keep them at home when they die. Now when they die we move them to a "funeral home" so that we can pretend they're at home.

LW: Right. I mean in the old days they used to have the casket, they used to have the viewing at home.

DK: And then they tell us they're just sleeping, they're not really gone. How can we deny death? It's such a part of life! It's just incredible to me. I think it's one of the most profound moments and we can be missing it half the time. There are two aspects I've noticed about dying at home. I've had patients in the hospital tell me, "If I can just get home to the things I love, to my cat, to my dog, to my neighbor, to my pictures, that's where my strength is. That's who I am. And that will help me recover." They find their healing strength at home. And then there are other patients who say, "I'm dying and it's time. Let me go home to the things I love. Let me die there, not surrounded by these four hospital walls."

BCM: How do you educate the families? This is such a cultural thing in our society. And it's such a hard thing. How do you help families even realize it is all right, that they can take care of someone at home? And then, of course, they've got to get through all of their own feelings of inadequacy and ineptitude. I learned all kinds of things that I never knew.

LW: Did you have nurses?

BCM: The last four nights we had hospice attendants and we had a hospice nurse come in every single day to check on Michael, but we learned how to do everything that you do to take care of someone because Michael was a helpless baby there at the end. And he was in a semicoma most of the time. Michael died at home with his extended family there. Our family experience was that we faced such trials within ourselves. We were afraid we would hurt him, or we would do it wrong, because we were not trained to take care of a dying person.

LW: Well, I was trained, but I was still not prepared.

BCM: None of us are trained to even take care of our babies, much less somebody who is dying.

DK: Did anyone train you in life? Life is terribly hard and so is death. I think some of the comfort is realizing that there are no great answers and there is no training and that whatever it will take you have within you.

BCM: What about the families, though, that feel unable to take care of their loved one? Their fear is just too great. How are we going to educate a populace that it is a viable, valuable alternative to have somebody die at home with good nursing care or even, if there's not a possibility of that, partial nursing care, or just the family taking care of that person?

LW: You know, it's hard for a family. It's really hard because in the hospital the nurses are so professional and so efficient and they are so starched. They bustle in and they bustle out, and they're so professional looking and you look at this in awe as a layperson and think, "How do they know how to do that?" So you are intimidated. And when you're around these nurses, these nurses do really want to help you, I think. Don't you? I know I always want to help the family. When I have a dying patient in the hospital, I spend a lot of time with that patient and whoever is there with him or her. Whether it be a spouse, a mother, a father, a brother, a sister, or a friend. I spend a lot of time with patients and their families teaching them things. I start teaching them immediately. If the Hickman catheter goes in, then I start teaching them immediately about Hickman care so that if the doctors tell them they're going to send the patient home with a Hickman, the family isn't saying, "Oh my God, do we have to learn this?" Because I've just been in there showing them. I start telling them about things like that. I start teaching them about nutrition. I start teaching them the importance of exercise. I start teaching them things about keeping their mind sane. I spend a lot of time with these patients and their families.

BCM: Where were you when so many of us needed you?

DK: And there's the whole emotional side to getting people ready. I think we all do the most we can do. Of course if you're lucky, you have a nurse who is there and can say to the family, "You know, I don't know right or wrong here and this person's going to die, but I'll be here. I'll see it through with you."

LW: Then there are the patients who end up going home by themselves, because their families are afraid to take them home with them. Sometimes the families see this atmosphere in the hospital and they're afraid. They're so afraid! They say, "We can never do this!"

BCM: Their own emotions are saying, "Help me, also!" When you are going through it all, you can hardly get up in the morning. You want to be there for the person, be there totally and unconditionally week after week. But then to have to learn new skills sometimes feels overwhelming, exhausting, impossible.

LW: The hospitals need to take a good look at that too and start teaching the families, the caregivers, whoever is going to be with that person until he dies. And the ones who are teaching the families need to understand what they are going through at this time. That's one of the things that the hospitals need to take a good look at any time there's a death and dying situation. I mean, my God, let's teach these patients everything that they need to know, but let's start out simply, so they don't feel like it's a teaching environment, because people learn more quickly that way.

DK: For this very reason we have a program at the nursing service that's seven weeks long. It's home nursing for nonprofessionals. It's a program for families and friends. It's great if someone doesn't have the resources of having nurses all the time and they need to learn more about how to care for the dying person. Or if they just want to learn more about how to be with someone who is dying. How afraid you're going to be when the situation isn't in control and you're not going to know what is a medical emergency from what isn't. And how to go through what you don't know to what you do know. The main thing we teach in that class is confidence. Because, I tell them in the beginning, the skills will be easy; once you learn when to panic and when not to panic, what's natural and what's part of the process, you'll feel so much more in control.

BCM: The bottom line in all of this is that we are in a process now, that death can, in a sense, be such a great teaching tool for all of us to learn how to be more complete human beings, how to deal with our own emotions and move through them, and our own fears.

DK: And we are moving to a new level of understanding.

LW: And we are still learning. We are always learning.

BCM: What is the most important thing you are learning?

DK: Learning how to live—through the dying, just learning how to live.

BCM: Just learning how to love. Understanding. Experiencing the love in all of this.

LW: Just experiencing the love.

When Someone You Love Has AIDS

The following excerpt is from the epilogue of When Someone You Love Has AIDS: A Book of Hope for Family and Friends, *a book I wrote about my son Michael and our shared journey through his life and death.*

When a child dies before his parents, no matter what his age, it violates the order of the universe. My son Michael died on July 14, 1986. He was twenty-eight years old.

He was surrounded by his loving family: his ex-step-mother, Nancy; me; and at various times during that last month of his life, his brothers, Bill, John, and Robert; his grandmother from Texas; and his father. Steve, his friend and therapist, was also there for him, as well as John, his roommate of several years. Friends called daily. Michael was also receiving devoted care from AIDS/Hospice workers, from Shanti counselors, and from his doctor. Yet although he was surrounded with the unconditional love and support he had asked for, still, Michael died.

He died at Nancy's house, a half block from his own apartment, as he had asked of us earlier, choosing to die at home rather than to be kept alive in the impersonality of the hospital. He made a conscious choice during that last month to let his deteriorating body go, and to let himself go to God. It was an agonizing time for all of us. And we will never be the same again.

For Michael did not "go gentle into that good night." To the very end, the human side of Michael fought for control, for mastery, for breath, for life—LIFE!—while the spiritual side of Michael, who had made his peace weeks before with death, wanted—begged, even—to leave the wasted body on the bed and escape gratefully into "that safe and peaceful place where Gee-Gee and Zacky are waiting for me." (Gee-Gee was Michael's great-grandmother and Zacky was Michael's nephew, who had died two years previously.)

How ironic that in the last weeks of Michael's life, we who had prayed so earnestly for Michael to live— "Michael, dear Michael, child of my heart. Don't die!"— now prayed through our tears for his swift release. Again and again the words rose from my heart, unspoken, "Michael, dear Michael, child of my heart. Let go! I release you to God, dear child."

For he was a child in those last few weeks. At times he was cross, fretful, angry, demanding, imperious. At times he was an eighty-pound baby, frightened, crying out for his two "mothers." At times he was a childlike spirit coming out of a comatose state to thank us all so politely for taking care of him.

Writing these words, I am reminded daily of that difficult time, when all I believed in about life, about death, about love, was put to the test. And if one sentence that I write can help another mother, another father, another brother or sister or grandmother, another lover or friend or health worker to understand the process of healing—yes, healing!—in the midst of the process called dying, then Michael's death will not have been in vain. I believe that just as there are alternatives in healing, like the ones Michael explored so diligently, and which resulted in a much longer life span for him than previously predicted, so there are alternatives available in the dying process itself. What we learned in those last few weeks of Michael's life can point the way for another family going through a similar situation.

For this is still a book of hope. This is, indeed, a book of love. And so I close my eyes and re-create the last weeks of Michael's life, not in despair, but in a spirit of hope; go back to that time when everything within me cried out for help in meeting the greatest crisis any mother can face, the death of her child.

Certain montages flicker before my eyes every time I close them, pictures that stand out with a clarity and intensity that match those last weeks the family went through. John, his brother from Texas, sleeping on the floor night after night, awake in an instant to lead Michael to the bathroom while he was still semiambulatory. John and I bathing Michael, and Michael's unself-conscious, childlike trust as he let the strong arms of his brother support him and help him with this most private of tasks.

I remember Bill, strong, reliable, tender-hearted Bill, Michael's oldest brother, faithfully transporting family members back and forth to be with Michael, and running errands for Michael for months. He and his family used to take Michael to Golden Gate Park to lie in the sun. They were there for him for months as loving helpers. And I remember Bill, near the end, consumed by grief both for his son, Zacky, remourning him, and for Michael. At one point he was unable to go up the stairs to Nancy's apartment to tend to Michael, and yet still, still, doing all he could for his brother. And I remember Bill holding me when Michael died.

I remember Nancy reaching out to me, standing shoulder to shoulder with me, holding hands at Michael's bedside when he had been comatose for fifteen hours. And I remember sleeping in a chaise lounge in Michael's room, counting the pauses between his breaths, willing him onward to where it would not hurt him to breathe. We looked down at this body, struggling to hold on to life. "Michael, dear Michael, child of our hearts. Let go!"

I remember Robert, my youngest son, calling daily, telling Michael again and again as we held the phone to his ear, "I love you, Spike." And I remember Michael's grandmother, walking into his room with a smile, dressed in a pastel dress, just off the plane from Texas, with all her love shining through her dear face, and Michael saying to her, "Oh, Grandmother, you're finally here. Now I know I am safe."

And I remember Nancy and I, with the help of the Shanti counselor, Karen, resolving old differences and falling into each other's arms saying, "I love you!"

The Shanti counselors and the AIDS/Hospice attendants who came the last few days of Michael's life cared both for Michael and for Nancy and me. They helped immeasurably, and their devotion and unselfish regard for all of us brings tears to my eyes even now. For every family caring for their loved one at home instead of in the hospital, I would beg you to contact both Shanti and Hospice. They serve unstintingly with love and practicality.

For there were times we did not think we could get through this last awesome task of caring for Michael at home. There were numbing fatigue, occasional outbursts of anger, grief so deep it could not be—and yet somehow was—borne, flashes of sheer terror. Am I strong enough, God, to be here for Michael? Am I strong enough to go through this valley, this shadowed place, with my heart wide open, with my arms wide open? Bathing Michael, lifting Michael, turning Michael, talking with Michael, listening to Michael, soothing Michael, medicating Michael. "Little bird, open your mouth," and his mouth would obey while the precious drops of morphine dropped in one by one, and then he would go off in a space so far from us that we were surprised each time he came back.

"He's apartment hunting," explained Frank, another Shanti counselor. "He goes out of his body and looks around and decides where he wants to be. But evidently," and he laughed, "he keeps coming back to Nancy's house because it's the most beautiful, comfortable place he can imagine."

"Let me sing to him while I'm taking care of him," said Sandy, one of the AIDS/Hospice attendants keeping the night vigil. "That will ease him so he won't be afraid." I looked into the room again and again that night, only to see this beautiful woman kneeling by Michael's bed, holding his hand, while he slept. Her soft lullaby words went on and on, while the candles guttered into dawn.

Within those nights there was time for me and, I trust, every one of us to revise our own feelings about death— time to go through each separate fear and anger and grief about Michael's dying. For although the dying process itself is a hard place inside you that seems to go on and on unbearably, unmercifully, and while watching your child die is the hardest task any of us will ever have to face, still, past the struggle there is death, merciful death, not to be dreaded, but to be welcomed. I said to myself again and again during those weeks, "Death is nothing to fear. Death is a kind friend."

The human spirit is resilient. The human spirit is love. Each of us had hourly opportunities to question and to experience the intensity of our feelings and the validity of our beliefs. We were challenged in each moment to be the love, the absolute, no-holds-barred, unconditional love that Michael had asked for. We were forced again and again to stretch ourselves to the limit of endurance, to the limit of love as we knew it.

And there were times when Michael himself was luminous. I remember an earlier visit, in June, when he sat by the fire in Nancy's living room, with a shawl around him, and we laughed and talked and were happy together.

For it was a joy to be in his presence and I want always to remember those moments, when Michael was more spirit than flesh, and yet, more alive, more here, more in the immediacy of the moment than I had ever seen him. We amazed ourselves at those times, at our laughter, at our spontaneous expressions of affection, at our own tenderness and vulnerability—and again, peacefulness—as Michael began to let go of his earthly form.

Michael had asked for three things to happen when he discovered he had AIDS.

He asked that everyone in his family be healed. Oh,

dearest Michael, that has come true! I remember Hedy, the head AIDS/Hospice nurse, leaning over him, whispering to him as she tried to find out what was holding Michael back from release during the last days of his life, what was holding him in this pattern of shuttling between the worlds of life and death, and understanding instinctively that he felt that he had not said good-bye to everyone. "Ah, Michael," she said gently, as he looked into her eyes and tried to make his wishes articulate. "All you have to do is say good-bye in your heart. And that person will know that you love and forgive him." An expression of peace passed over Michael's face and he fell asleep.

The second thing that Michael had asked for was to be surrounded by unconditional love. During the last years of his life, everyone he knew cared deeply about him, from his workmates to his friends, to the helpers that attended him, to every member of his family. No one experienced more love than Michael did up to the last moments of his life. And that love continues even now.

The third thing that Michael had asked for was to be able to do the work that was his to do. When I first began writing this story of Michael's journey through AIDS, he was aflame with enthusiasm. He envisioned himself reaching out to others who had AIDS. He saw himself telling his story, unafraid, risking his self through telling the truth about his illness. More importantly, he wanted to share his deepest self in courage and in love. He talked often about the awakening that AIDS had brought into his life, the 180-degree turnaround that had led him into a deepening relationship with God. He wanted to make a difference in the world.

"AIDS is a gift. AIDS has removed the barriers between me and other people. AIDS is the catalyst that has taught me how to love."

He believed at the time that he would live. I believed this, too. In fact, there was a time when Michael thought himself to be a failure because his physical body was obviously deteriorating, despite all his efforts to heal himself within and without by every means available to him at that time. This trap of spiritual pride, wherein you are "good" if you demonstrate health and "bad," "wrong," or a "failure," if the body does not follow your commands, was a hard lesson for Michael to learn. He went through a time of profound anguish, continually seeking to understand, continually seeking peace at a deeper level, and finally, I trust, letting go of the belief that insisted that healing was limited to the physical body and that not healing meant failure.

"Facts are the enemy of Truth," said Don Quixote. This statement has helped me to understand that Michael's healing was accomplished. It is true that his physical body, after more than two years with the AIDS diagnosis, did, in fact, consume itself. And it is equally true that Michael will live forever—in our hearts, in our minds, in our souls.

I like to think that Michael did, indeed, get his last wish—that of making a difference in the world through telling his story with courage and love.

I remember one of the nights I was sleeping in his room, with the lamp turned down so low that there were only shadows in the room, except for the light that fell upon Michael. Around midnight, dozing in and out of a fretful sleep, the little voice came from the bed. "Mama, Mama," and I roused myself. After I had tended to his physical needs and kissed him and smoothed his hair back from his childlike, cadaverous face, he gestured for the legal pad and pen we used to write down his medications. It was extremely hard for Michael to speak at this point. The Kaposi's sarcoma had taken over the roof of his mouth and his throat so that he could not eat, could barely swallow. He spoke slowly, croakily, urgently.

"Write . . . this . . . down, . . . Mama. . . . Write . . . this . . . down."

I obediently took the pad and pen and waited, poised. Michael often dictated his requests to us, and we laughingly said that he would stay in control through his dictation process until his last breath.

I understood immediately that Michael's mind was wandering and that he thought I was still writing the book about his life. He had often questioned me in the last few weeks about some minor points in the book, chiefly those that dealt with the changes that had taken place within him both physically and emotionally, since the book had first been published in an earlier edition.

"Write this down, Mama. . . . Now. . . . Write this down."

He dictated slowly, with long pauses between words.

"I, Michael, . . . am peaceful now. . . . Because I am not . . . yelling at my mother anymore. . . . Because I love and . . . appreciate her so."

I waited, tears streaming down my face, for more. What did Michael have to say that was so urgent that it could bring him back to coherency, however briefly, with such urgency? What words were there to leave the world to remember him by?

But there was only silence.

I touched Michael's face. He was sleeping peacefully. All trace of tension was gone from his face. I did not know it then, but except for a few disconnected phrases, Michael would not speak coherently again.

Yet in that early morning moment, Michael told me what I most needed to hear. That he was peaceful. That his struggle was over. And that he loved me. His message was not for the whole world. And yet I share it with you now. "I love you." As he did us all.

I love you too, Michael. And I always will. Sleep, little one. You are safe. It's only change. Go forward in love.

I Want to Go Home

Mary Schramski wrote movingly of her reconciliation with her father, her caregiving, and his remission from cancer in an earlier part of this book. Several years later the cancer returned. Mary then moved her father into her home for the remaining eight months of his life. Portions of this story appeared in a slightly different form in Personal Transformation *magazine, Winter 1994.*

My father, always the Southern gentleman, asked me to bring his guests something to eat or drink. His eyes looked beyond me as I studied his gaunt face, the high cheekbones and prominent nose protruding even further because of his weight loss, the folds of the pillow forming a halo around his head. Alone in the back bedroom of my home, my father lay in the hospital bed that had been ordered for him a month earlier.

"Dad, are you sure you don't want something?" I asked. He had not eaten anything in over three weeks, only taking small sips of water to moisten his mouth, but every day, five or six times, I offered him food. My hope for his life and recovery died a very slow death. His big brown eyes searched my face and he smiled slightly.

"No, but get everyone else whatever they want, honey."

Automatically, I glanced around the room. Everyone else? His sincere look told me not to doubt what he was saying, and even though his cancer had rendered him helpless, his Southern upbringing kicked into gear and he played the good host.

"Dad, who are these people you want me to get something for?"

"I don't know them." He shrugged, not worried.

"Where are they?"

"They're right here beside you." He paused, looking over my shoulder, then closed his eyes. Fatigue was his friend now, slipping him into a more gentle, painless sphere.

I glanced around again, hoping to catch a look at my father's newfound friends. I could not see the people he talked to me about. I felt that this was a sign my father would probably die soon.

All my life I had heard from relatives, and read, that when people are dying, they see people, spirits from the other side who come to guide the dying, helping to make their transition easier. I had often doubted those tales, never experiencing or seeing them myself. And now my father, whom I trusted and loved, was asking me to get his spiritual visitors refreshments.

It had been a long road for us. A few years ago the doctors diagnosed Dad's backache as terminal cancer. Now he was fighting the final stages. My husband and I had made a commitment to Dad. We would care for him in our home. With the help of hospice, we would fight the battle with him. We all struggled, watching a vital man cut down by cancer, thin slices of human dignity taken away day after day.

Sheets of light showered his bedroom. Where were these people my father was seeing? When my father said something, it was believable. Not a man of frivolity, he had flown airplanes for thirty-six years and plotted courses that never varied. Now there were people surrounding him who he did not know but he was not afraid. His graciousness touched my heart. He was so ill yet he thought of others, helping me realize even in the face of death that we are not alone.

This was a message to me. My kind father was leaving and I needed to let go. We had fought for so long, thinking many times that we could win this battle with cancer. Now I needed to realize there wasn't a war.

The day after his invisible visitors, my father's health aide from hospice made her usual house call. Dad loved Julia and trusted her. He often called her Julia Child, his sense of humor never leaving him, as she diligently helped him with his bath.

Checking to see if Julia needed any help, I knocked on the bedroom door and stuck my head in. She and my father, who sat on the edge of his bed, stared at me.

"Your father, he wants to take a shower," Julia stated in her lyrical African accent. My father had refused showers for over a month because of his fatigue, and Julia had dutifully prepared sponge baths for him.

"Do you think you can get him in the shower, Julia? I can help you." Her muscular body was more than capable of handling my father, his weight now down to just under a hundred pounds. My voice grew squeaky with hope. We had been entrapped in an emotional death maze for so long, just hearing my father say he wanted to take a shower sent my mind reeling. At that moment I didn't care what the doctors or hospice said. Surely if my father wanted a shower, he was not going to die. The three of us became a tableau of hope facing a miracle.

"We'll try, right, Mr. Hauser?" Julia encouraged. Dad looked up at me, his haunting limpid eyes scanning my face.

"I'm going home, honey," he stated matter-of-factly, not blinking, waiting for my response.

"You're going home?" I asked, my hopes bounding again.

"I've got to go home," he answered, looking confused at my question. Over the months I had become the mother in a way, feeding him, helping him in and out of bed, and for the last three weeks even changing him. I knew my father. This elegant Southern gentleman wasn't going anywhere without a shower.

"I think that's a great idea, Dad. Go home, it's time. Julia will help you get cleaned up so you can go." The words flowed easily out of my mouth even as I realized my father was talking about dying.

"When shall I go?" His question stunned me. How could I play God, telling him when to die? Thankfully a quiet strength came over me.

"Dad, you go home when you want to. You have to choose the time. But Dad, will you come back and visit me?" I couldn't give my father permission to die without some promise I would see him again.

"Yes, I will," he answered.

The transformational moment ended and Julia tried to get my father into the shower, but it proved impossible. He was too weak. After a sponge bath, he drifted into a peaceful sleep. The next day, Saturday, he progressed into a semicoma, dying Sunday morning at 3:00 A.M.

Four days later, at 2:30 A.M., my father kept his promise to me by appearing in my bedroom. Dad woke me with a hug. I felt the pressure of his familiar embrace against my shoulder as he knelt over my bed. It was dark in the room, but I knew it was he. Dressed in a brown robe, a hood covering his head, monk-like, he communicated the thought, "Now can I do the dishes?" The communication was clear and the impression strong. Even though my husband was gone on a business trip, I was not afraid. I felt great joy just being with Dad again.

My father left just as quickly as he had drifted in and I lay in bed, savoring the experience. The hug had meant so much. During the last few months of his illness, Dad and I hugged four or five times a day. I would hug him and tell him I loved him. He would respond in kind and as his illness progressed, the hugs grew more important to both of us. A profound love surrounded us, pure and caring, a father and daughter struggling through life and facing death together.

"Now can I do the dishes?" Not a very earth-shattering message, but it contained a special meaning for me. Before cancer shattered his life and took away his strength, I did the cooking and my dad and I would banter every night about the cleanup. He wanted to do the dishes, but there was a problem he didn't know about. When my father cleaned the kitchen, he ran a lot of water. My husband, a conservative man, would roll his eyes at me as the water in the kitchen ran and ran, and I would shrug my shoulders. My father was oblivious to this pantomime. Every night I would offer to wash the dishes, but would give in knowing it made my dad feel useful.

If anyone would keep a promise, it would be Dad. He was a man of his word. The message he brought me wasn't profound, nothing about the mystery of life and death, but it is mine. Now I know, without doubt, my father didn't die. He just went home, leaving his tired, sick body behind.

Dad was a stable, forthright person. He never criticized, never judged, and took most things in stride. His fear of his illness and death overwhelmed him at times and it forced me to look for answers for myself. My father's journey to death changed me. My fears of illness, life, death, and the unknown are gone. There are many things I don't understand, but I now trust in what I cannot see, as my father trusted his unknown visitors.

My family and friends tell me how lucky my father was to have such a devoted daughter to take care of him. I never felt he was the lucky one to have me. I am the blessed one. I was given the chance to look at life and death close up and open my heart to both.

Letting Go

Every person's death is unique, as every person is unique. And the loved ones who wait and watch with them, the loved ones who see the caregiving through to its very end, often seem to come to a place of prayer that is different from the "God help me! or "God help my loved one to live and be well!" exhortations that formed the basis for fervent prayer at an earlier time. When this does not happen, when all our prayers are for the singular outcome we envision, I believe it is more difficult for our loved ones to let go, to be released from the suffering, and to go on. I remember when my two cousins' father died, in his mideighties, after years of being cared for by his wife. She collapsed as the primary caregiver and was rushed to the hospital and then into a small-town nursing home. My two cousins moved their father into their two homes. He would spend five days at one home, while the other cousin worked, then be moved on the weekend to that cousin's home. They enlisted the help of one of their husbands and a strong, burly son, because to lift this skeletal man, and fold his six-foot frame into a car or wheelchair or move him from bed to couch was a herculean job.

It was a time of great travail for all, and yet a bonding occurred between the two previously estranged cousins. They were working together puposefully, in order to do what had to be done.

One cousin told me later that even though it was only for two months, the experience was the most harrowing one she had ever gone through, and she would have nightmares the rest of her life remembering her father's moans and cries of help as he struggled to let go.

At her father's funeral, another family member came up to us as we all stood talking afterward. She struggled to find some word of condolence for my two cousins. "I am so sorry for both of you in this tragic loss. God has ways we know not of," she said, or something to that effect, and followed with, "there are no words for such a loss as yours." My cousins answered her firmly and in unison. "The word we have is 'Rejoice!' Rejoice that our father is relieved of his terrible agony and has gone onward to a better place." I have never forgotten those words.

A nurse in a care facility told me once that one of the ironic messages of working in a nursing home, and one of the saddest, according to her, is when the family is divided. "You will see families praying at the bedside of their loved one, and that is, of course, heartwarming. At least the person is loved and will not die alone. But often some of the family are insistent on the ill person living, of conforming to their idea of what is best for their loved one. Why, I have seen families pray a parent out of a coma," she exclaimed, "when all the while, you know that the aged, terminally ill person just wants to let go peacefully, and escape from a body they have outworn. Sometimes I can tell that the people who pray for their loved one to live are very afraid of loss and death. Maybe they think that by the sheer magnitude and volume of their prayers, God will hear them and spare their loved one. But spare them for what? Increasing pain, debilitation, and mental confusion? Sometimes the one who is doing the bulk of the caregiving is the most silent. One time I swear I saw the eyelids of a comatose woman move from side to side, as one part of the family prayed on one side of the bed, and on the other side, another family member sat silent, holding her hand. I knew without a shadow of a doubt that the ill person was going from side to side in her mind, matching her eye movements, deciding whether to stay or to go."

This scenario is more common than you may think. But everyone has to let go eventually, and a prayer that asks for only one outcome, an earthly outcome, is in my opinion the cruelest and most misguided prayer of all.

Perhaps you are not a praying person. My father, who served in World War II, often used the old adage, "There are no atheists in foxholes." In my observation, caregivers and their loved ones, whatever their previous religious ideas, turn in their trouble, to some force greater than their situation, and ask for help. And as the caregiving progresses, they ask for more and more help. A strong faith in God can get you through when nothing else seems to. Yet when our prayers fail us, or seem to, then what do we do? Do we turn away? Do we feel that we have been abandoned by God? Every childhood image of God may come back to haunt us. We may struggle to believe, when the evidence before our eyes is so overwhelmingly tragic. It may take some time, both during the caregiving and after the caregiving, for our basic faith to be restored. For we are changed by the journey. Our belief system is altered. We have been through the fire. We will never be the same again.

When people ask me how they can go on when their prayers have not been answered, I have no easy answer. The only thing I can say is that by praying for the highest good for all concerned, for the highest good of the ill person, for the highest good in the situation, for the highest and best good for the heart of each family member, then, and then only, can we begin to let go. And we can begin to let our loved one go. A prayer of release can be a courageous blessing. "Not my will, but Thine, be done." We pray then for our own acceptance, our own release as well. We have shared the pain of our loved one's journey. There comes a time, whatever it takes within us, for us to let go. For us to let our loved one go. It is the final and most unselfish act we can do. We ask for peace for our loved one, and for his or her passing. We ask for peace for ourselves. And we accept.

After the Caregiving

The Continuity of Life

The wise and knowing part, vastly in tune with life, brings its wisdom to mother/grandmother and says, "This is the stuff character is made of. . . ."

Once life is conceived, its entire rhythm is to be experienced. Breathe deeply; learn to flow with it. The great pain of your labor will be followed by the incredible beauty and joy of new life.

The age-old wisdom comes to us from every direction. Yesterday I buried my daughter and grandchild. Happily, today a man tells me of the birth of a new child and I smile at him with love. He has thus assured me of the continuity of life.

—REVEREND CAROL W. PARRISH-HARRA

After the Caregiving

Grieve fully
Take lots of walks
Join a support group
Join an exercise class
Join a meditation class
Ease slowly back into work or family responsibilities
Catch up on your sleep
Clean out your closets
Take a vacation
Plan one day a week just for creativity and joy
Renew old friendships
Make new friends
Follow a good nutrition plan
Read lots of inspiring books
Plant a garden
Be good to yourself

Grief Recovery: The Stepping Stones

The Decision to Ask for Help
The Willingness to Shatter
The Hope to Find a Way Through
The Honesty to Look Within
The Patience to Stick with the Process
The Trust to Keep Open
The Gratitude to Pass It On

Exercise as a Tool of Power

I have never known anyone who was a long-term caregiver who didn't need exercise. No, not the kind that comes of physically lifting and bathing and caring for a loved one. Or from the endless round of meals and housekeeping and all the daily chores of existence that make caregiving exhausting, no matter how long the experience.

After the caregiving, most caregivers are too tired to even think about themselves, much less in terms of formal physical exercise. Many have bypassed vanity in favor of instant practicality, and their own health in favor of the seemingly endless needs of the patient that they tend.

Physical and emotional collapse is often imminent. Indeed, many sick people outlive their primary caregivers.

It doesn't have to be that way. Perhaps you have neglected yourself and your needs for so long that your body is rusty and your emotions numb. Your concentrated focus has been on others for so long that you may have forgotten what it feels like to move for the pure joy of movement. To move for *you* and for *your* health. It's not too late. Here is a prescription for caregivers. Whether you can begin during the caregiving or must wait, for needs' sake, until after the caregiving is over, exercise as a tool of power can be an integral part of your own recovery.

Every type of exercise, as well as each specific exercise engaged in, creates a dynamic tension of stress (positive stress), of muscles working together or against each other, of accelerated circulation and respiration. Physical exercise stirs up the stagnant places within the body and helps to release dead cells, excess water, excess pounds and inches, and firms, tones, and strengthens our bodies throughout their various activities. Physical exercise awakens the body to its own strength, its own potential, its capacity for renewal.

It has been said that many of us are dead from the neck down. Stiffness of joints can indicate stiff, hard, resistant attitudes toward change. By moving the body more, the flow of energy begins to operate. Stir up your body and you may rid yourself of aches and pains. Better yet, as you contact the stronger you within and release great blocks of tension, you free energy. Tension is only trapped energy. As you release it, you become stronger in a positive, life-giving way. Your image of yourself begins to change.

Change creates change. The stagnant energies and the tense, tight crystallizations within are dissolved and dissipated. Just as the physical toxins pour out of you in the form of cleansing perspiration when you exercise, so do the psychological toxins flow out of you. They are released naturally as your energy is released.

As always, mind, body, and emotions work together. As you rid yourself of all that you do not want, you lay hold of health and strength and wholeness, all the qualities that you do want. And you incorporate these qualities into your system in a dynamic way as you move. You tune in to your own self. You tune in to your own power and potential. You begin to know, to express, and to respect your own, unique, beautiful body.

When in doubt, when tired, when sleepy, when irritated, tense, or frustrated, don't just sit there. Move! If you are grieving, move. (A friend of mine told me that she ran her grief away.) If you are angry at loss, move. If you are in despair, move. For movement creates flow. Movement stirs up the circulation, the respiration, the digestion. Movement stirs up the emotions as well, brings them to the surface to be faced, felt, cleansed, and released from deep within you. Any kind of movement you choose at first will do. But move! Stretch! Bend! Shake your legs and arms! Jump in place, dance, walk, jog. You can even play. Play! Now that's a thought. Something you probably haven't done for years. Along with the movement, whatever form it takes, engage your breathing. Long, deep breaths help you to release the emotions, and, paradoxically, calm and relax the body as well.

Sometimes what is simplest works the best. The decision to use exercise as a part of your healing after the caregiving is a decision you make for yourself, for your own health, for your own joy, for your own recovery from loss. It will be the first of many good decisions you will make for yourself after the caregiving. Do it for yourself. Begin now.

The Train Through Life and Death

Helen Cook is a great-grandmother from Texas whose insights on grieving through the generations, what she calls "the train through life and death," have a poignancy and wisdom distilled from years of living. Her life is a gift to me and to all who know her. She wrote this story when she was seventy years old.

Today I cried. I needed those tears. I needed to grieve for my grandson who died some years ago. I had not been able to cry, and that left me tied into a hard knot. I felt that I had been holding my breath for so long that my body was stiff and unyielding, afraid to let go and let the tears wash away the grief, the anguish, the loneliness, the guilt—all the hurting feelings that beset us when we lose someone we love.

My grandson Michael died of AIDS, and I watched his life prolonged beyond reason with suffering. I wanted to gather him up into my arms like a little child, and hold him against all hurt, all pain, all uncertainty in his mind. But all I could do was to help him pass the hours and the days with stories of the years when he was a young boy and relive the memories we had of happy times together. He would go back to those years over and over, so we relived them together, so he could forget the dreadful present.

I cried for my sisters today too. Both dead and gone, as are my brother, my father, my mother, my husband as well. Dorothy, my oldest sister, was always so much fun, until she got sick. She used to ride motorcycles and loved to dance. She was so much wilder than I ever was. I was always the timid one. My younger sister, Betty, was an alcoholic, and we had a hard time understanding each other during the last ten years of her life. In my inner strength and zeal, I could not imagine what could lead anyone to destroy her body and her mind with alcohol. I know I do not truly understand this disease, and I felt guilty because I could not fill her great need for someone to be beside her and encourage her. Yet, like so many of us, she really wanted to be alone. It bothered her to have a "watchdog" monitoring her every act. I am glad to say that we shared many weekends of fun and companionship during the past few years, as we visited and played lots of card games, and enjoyed each other more than we ever had in years past. Yet I could not cry for Betty when she died.

It seems to be always the past that helps us to bear the troubles and sorrows of the present. So I took to my past to explain some of my inability to shed tears.

When asked at seventy to think back on how I faced grief in my lifetime, I must go back to the first funeral that I remember. Picture, if you will, a small active girl of about seven years, black hair in a Dutch bob. She is wearing a maroon velveteen dress trimmed with braid, and her sister

Dorothy, a few years older, wears an identical dress in dark green. They are too warm for the early spring day, but the dresses were gifts brought from Chicago by the grandfather who is being buried today. I do not quite understand when I see a great-aunt suddenly burst into tears and just as suddenly avert her face and stiffen her narrow shoulders as she silently wipes her face on a lace-edged handkerchief. The funeral itself is an innovation in our lives, and the arrival at the old country cemetery a whole new adventure.

I do not know my grandfather very well, for he does not live with my grandmother; but the feelings I can sense in my mother and her sister, the aunts and uncles who are my grandfather's children, as hard as that is to imagine, all combine to fill me with an urge to cry as my mother is crying. But my grandmother is standing behind me, her long fingers steady on my shoulders. When I look up at her, I cannot find the soft twinkle in her eyes that always met mine. Today, she stares across the cemetery, looking away from all that is going on, her face as stony as the headstones around us. I want to cry out, but those fingers hold me still, captured by her stony grief.

I was only in my late thirties when I lost my husband. Dare I go back to that time, so far away, to resurrect that other lifetime? It is as if forgetting that time in my life will make the pain go away. John was seven years older than me, and we met when I was only fourteen, but waited to be married until three days before I became eighteen. He spoiled me, loved me, left me a legacy of a gentle man, the father of my three daughters. When he died after a long illness, I felt pressured by all I had to do, to keep the funeral plans, sleeping arrangements, meals, and baby-sitting all coordinated for that week, so that none of the family and friends would have to worry about anything. It was as if I grabbed all those plans and made them mine, because I was so good at details. I was not good at loss and grieving. I had cried all my tears the year before when the doctor told me that John could not live out the year, possibly only three or four months. That first night, I buried John several times, grieving and picking out pallbearers and telling the children. The night was filled with all my weeping, so that the next morning and for more than another year, I was able to face and take care of the mundane part of my life, putting aside the grief.

Sometimes I can't remember how he looked or the way his voice sounded, and I panic! And then, the few times he has come to me in dreams, we have neither of us become any older. His picture on the dresser in my bedroom faces me, his eyes so warm and brown, crinkling at the corners, his smile, those perfect teeth, his voice enclosing me in safety and love. But I feel that must have been in another lifetime. We exist together only in memories, only in the past. He is just waiting for me. We'll be together again someday. Maybe soon.

I am ruled in many ways by the past. As with Michael and my husband: we shared memories that made grief bearable, although sometimes unexpressed.

With my mother, it was different. I believe we were more like twins than mother and daughter. We had a special affinity between us. So many of our feelings, thoughts, and beliefs were the same. Many times we knew instinctively what the other was thinking or was going to say. We could sit in companionable silence, tuned in to the same wavelength of thoughts. Losing her to death was like a part of me dying.

On a hot summer night after she died, I could hear the telephone ringing and ringing next door in my mother's empty house. I could cover my ears and sob into my pillow, but the ringing would still be there inside my head. By rigidly suiting my manner to that of the generations before me, I could keep my chin up and my eyes dry among others. Yet every night, alone, my heart would continue breaking.

One cold winter evening, arriving home in the early dark, a great wave of grief enveloped me as I groped for the garage door, in the shadow of the empty house next door. My mother had always turned on her backyard light for me and tapped on her back room window to let me know she was watching out for my safety. I knew, then, that she had been with me in so many ways that I could never lose her again, although the hurt will always be there. It is the little things, the sudden ways that life's events remind us of the great love we had, that makes us want to run to our mother's arms, and be a child once more, so snug, so safe.

On one Thanksgiving Day, a holiday my mother always loved, I was missing her warmth and her humor and her little laugh. And I recalled so many drives we had made up to that little north Texas town to visit the two great-aunts. And while I thought about it, I was certain my mother was having Thanksgiving dinner with the aunts, in heaven, laughing and talking and enjoying one another as they always did.

Traditions in the holidays go on as usual. I still carefully unwrap the tiny wax turkeys and Indians and Pilgrims to grace the Thanksgiving table, at whichever house we have gathered that year. The wrappings are threadbare and falling apart, just an old white grocery sack I could replace easily with a new strong one. But this sack is special. This one has my mother's distinctive, almost unreadable handwriting on it, indicating that Indians and Pilgrims dwell within.

Sometimes I see a glimpse of our whole family, from its earliest years, as in a railroad station, figures only dimly seen and unrecognizable in the mist and shadows. But there is a constant movement as trains come and go: passengers getting off trains, others getting on. The new babies are handed off the train to eager waiting arms; those who are leaving are getting on the train. Yet there is no rush. All know where they are going, at their appointed time. It is a joy to see a new young face. It is doubly a joy to get on the train and greet an old familiar one.

How close we are to those others who precede us into heaven! There are cords between us, sensitive and unseen, yet stronger than death, stronger than life itself, as strong as love and faith.

Yet I have faced grief so many times and have seldom been granted the blessing of tears. I am still that child standing in the winds of a country cemetery. There are silent, stern faces above and around me; my grandmother's strong restraining hands on my shoulders keep me wrapped in a wall of coldness against death. I have seldom been able to break down that barrier.

I wish they had let me cry. I wish they had told me it was all right. Nevertheless, today I cried. I cried for me.

A Minister Looks at Stages of Loss

BY REVEREND MARGIE ANN NICOLA, D.D.

In observing those who are "left behind," I have found there is a recognizable evolution of grief. Below, I outline some of the stages of grief many people experience, and include suggestions for coping with these feelings.

DENIAL OF LOSS

"I should not grieve, for God needs him more than I do." "She's gone on to her good so I'm okay." "We were together for so many years, I must be grateful for what I had." "I'm just feeling sorry for myself if I feel bad." And on and on.

When we love, we may experience loss. The pain of loss is a real and powerful experience. Grieving is necessary. To reenter the mainstream of life, we must allow ourselves to feel the feelings so that we can release them. The pain of loss is normal and natural.

GUILT OVER UNFINISHED BUSINESS

"If I could have just said I was sorry. . . ." "If she would have forgiven me. . . ." "I should have visited more." "I should have been more loving."

Because I believe death is merely moving into another dimension of living, I encourage those left behind to write a letter to the friend or loved one who has just died, or in their mind to express the feelings and say the words that were not shared. I believe that in God there is no time and space, therefore the words and feelings are received and a healing takes place.

GUILT FOR FEELING "THEY FINALLY DIED"

We may feel a sense of relief when someone we love dies. This experience usually follows a long illness that has placed stress on the family left behind. Or perhaps the deceased was a controller and had made the bereaved's life miserable.

If we will deal with our feelings honestly rather than burying or denying them, we will move through them faster and with less pain.

ANGER WITH THE PERSON FOR DYING

This happens often and is seldom talked about. Anger usually occurs with the death of a spouse or parent. There is a sense of betrayal and abandonment. This is a natural reaction to the loss.

Again, if we do not fight or deny this feeling, it will pass. The anger is a result of fear. Involvement in life will alleviate the fear and anger.

DEPRESSION

This can follow any of the previous stages. Often it occurs because the bereaved stops in the middle of a process and does not move on to his or her next step in grieving and returning to life.

Seek professional and spiritual help. The longer we allow ourselves to be depressed, the more difficult it is to release it. Depression is a result of immobility of thought and activity. Find something in life to capture your mind and imagination.

THE SENSE OF LOSS

This is a natural, normal emotional separation. This stage may encompass some or all of the above stages. Allow emotions to surface and then move on through the experience. Accept the pain and know that it will diminish and recede.

A belief system that provides a strong foundation, a comforting reassurance that all is well in spite of the loss, creates the space in which we can allow ourselves to understand that pain and loss are a part of living. We are more than our pain and more than our loss.

ANNIVERSARIES

Grief resurfaces on the anniversaries of the death and special events that had been shared, such as family gatherings.

Again, rather than withdrawing from the experience, participate both in the event and in the remembrance. This is very normal and natural.

As a counselor, I see my function as recognizing which stage of grief counselees are in and assisting them to move through the process and reenter their everyday activities as quickly and easily as possible. Compassion rather than sympathy, encouragement rather than commiseration, seem to be the best supports I can offer.

I say to each person grieving, when you add up all your life experiences, even the painful ones, they have created the opportunity for you to become strong in mind and forced you to seek higher wisdom and guidance.

In spite of every wound you have been dealt, you have not been destroyed, and the pain you have experienced may have been the driving force for you to turn to a higher power.

Until we give up our belief that pain should be avoided at all costs, and we allow ourselves to go through the pain, we will never face the past, forgive it, accept it, and love it. The past represents Life, and we cannot deny Life and still expect to enjoy what Life has to give us.

Symptoms of Loss

Deborah Roth, of the Center for Help in Time of Loss, contributed this from her book Stepping Stones to Grief Recovery.

Most people who suffer a loss may find themselves going through any of the following experiences:

- Feeling tightness in the throat or heaviness in the chest. Having an empty feeling in their stomach and losing their appetite.
- Feeling restless and looking for activity but finding it difficult to concentrate.
- Feeling as though the loss isn't real, that it didn't happen.
- Sensing the loved one's presence, such as finding themselves expecting the person to walk in the door at the usual time, hearing their voice, or seeing their face.
- Wandering aimlessly and forgetting or not finishing things they've started to do around the house.
- Having difficulty sleeping, and dreaming of their loved one frequently.
- Experiencing an intense preoccupation with the life of the deceased.
- Assuming mannerisms or traits of their loved one.
- Feeling guilty or angry over things that happened or didn't happen in the relationship with the deceased.
- Feeling intensely angry at the loved one for leaving them.
- Feeling as though they need to take care of other people who seem uncomfortable around them by politely not talking about their feelings of loss.
- Needing to tell, retell, and remember things about the loved one and the experience of their death.
- Feeling mood changes over the slightest things.
- Crying at unexpected times.

These are all natural and normal grief responses and must be experienced fully in order to heal and go forward.

Blest Are the Sorrowing: They Shall Be Consoled

This poem is reprinted from Being Human in the Face of Death. *Its authorship is unknown.*

And what does it mean to mourn?
I asked the multitude.
And an old man stepped forward.

To mourn, he said, is to be given a second heart.
It is to care so deeply
that you show your ache in person.

To mourn is to be unashamed of tears.
It is to be healed
and broken
and built-up all in the same moment.

Blessed are you if you can minister to others
with a heart that feels
with a heart that hurts
with a heart that loves
and blessed are you if you can minister to others
with a heart that serves
and a heart that sees the need before it's spoken.

To mourn is to forget yourself for a moment and get
    lost
in someone else's pain
and then,
to find yourself
in the very act of getting lost.

*To mourn is to be an expert
in the miracle
of being careful with another's pain.*

*It is to be full of the willingness
of forever reaching out to
and picking up
and holding carefully
those who hurt.*

*To mourn is to sing with the dying
and to be healed
by the song
and the death.*

Throwing Stones

I wrote this after a series of devastating losses in my life, and when I was only halfway through my caregiver journey with my mother. It is the story audiences most request when I do readings. It is reprinted here with gratitude to New World Library/Wildcat Canyon Press, where it first appeared in my book Soulwork: Clearing the Mind, Opening the Heart, Replenishing the Spirit.

At a time in my life when despair seemed the order of the day and my teeth ground in frustration at every passing sling and arrow, I talked to a friend of mine who had weathered, with grace and courage, some of the same challenges that I was going through. I asked her what to do.

"Throw stones," she advised me.

"What?"

"It's an exercise, a ritual, an exorcism if you will," she

said. Since my friend is practical, tough, and clearheaded, I swallowed my skepticism and asked for details.

"It's called the resentment exercise," she explained, "and I'll share it with you, but you must promise to do all the steps involved. Just thinking about it isn't enough."

"Why?" I asked again.

"Because the mind needs concrete evidence to re-arrange its patterns, and the emotions need motion in order to do the same."

I dutifully promised.

It was like a recipe. It went like this:

Write down on a piece of paper all—all!—the frustra-tions and resentments you are filled with, past and present, trivial or catastrophic.

"*All?*" I inquired again in disbelief.

"Well," she said, "the first time I did this exercise, I couldn't bear to write down my feelings about my father's stroke, my mother's violent, uncontrollable Alzheimer's, or the book project that fell through after months of work." (She is a writer too.) "Write down most of your resent-ments," she said. "You can tackle the major issues later, in a month or two, after you lighten the load."

It definitely needed lightening. But in my curious, stub-born fashion, my essential nature got the better of me, and I included everything on my list. I counted twenty-one hurts, angers, fears. How could anyone hold twenty-one resentments over the years? I told you I included every-thing.

"Number the resentments," advised my friend, "and then go to the store and buy a marking pen."

I did as I was told.

"Now," she said, "gather stones."

"What?"

"Gather stones. Go out to the country or a park and gather stones." I didn't need to ask how many.

"Yes," she affirmed. "One stone for each numbered resentment on your list. Mark each stone with a corresponding number. Then," she said, "you'll be ready. You'll be ready to throw your stones."

The day was stormy when I began to gather my stones, my list and marking pen clutched in my hand. I gathered them by color, weight, size, configuration. Not unlike, I reflected, the individual resentments on my list. I felt both foolish and mysterious. I was an ancient priestess gathering gifts to assuage the fates. The situation portended good.

Here was a rock for heartbreak—sharp and jagged with gray-blue veins running through it. Here was a heavy, slimy, misshapen stone. I knew what number I would write on it. Here were small stones of triviality. Here were stones of dark and deep. I gathered them all, twenty-one stones, each one discrete and different, each one a problem unresolved, each one an emotional universe.

I sat on the curb above the park, there where the sere and wintry grass hugged a ravine full of brush. I sorted my stones. I marked my stones, white ink on dark rock. I consulted my list. I looked everywhere around me. There was no one watching. Only me and my stones.

Then, slowly, carefully, ceremoniously, I began to throw my stones into the ravine, whispering their messsages after them as they skidded down the hill. When I was finished, even the wind was still. There was only the echo of my voice on the air and the sound of my breath, gritty as gravel, in my throat. I tore up the written list and scattered its strips into the ravine as well.

"No more," I said. "Done." I might have said more. But I noticed then that the gravel in my throat was gone. As was the heaviness in my gut. As was the pain in my right side that had plagued me with its insistent, incessant throbbing. As was the stone that had heretofore pierced my heart. I was lighter. I was clear. I was empty.

I called my friend. I told her about throwing stones. "I may have to repeat the experience in a few months," I told her. "There may be more."

"Of course," she said. "There's bound to be more." Her mother had just died, without recognizing the face of the daughter who had cared for her.

I offered to come to her area of the country to be with her. "We could," I ventured, "throw stones together."

She began to cry. "Hurry," she said to me. "Bring stones. Bring lots and lots of stones."

My Mother Is More Peaceful Now

My mother is more peaceful now. She has been moved to a small Episcopal facility, equidistant between my sister's house and mine. Shared care. Continuing care. I travel fifty minutes each way to see her, two hours there, fifty minutes home. Four hours, many days. Five years.

She is happier there. She knows who I am, although she introduces me sometimes to staff and residents alike as "this is my mother."

But she is more peaceful now. There are still hallucinations, there are still floods of tears, there is still swift anger and a bewildering, unreasoning fear that grips her and makes her words incoherent. In the midst of her struggle to communicate with me, she will grip my hand and let the words spill out over me like a flood, hoping that her intent will make them comprehensible. Sometimes she is lucid.

She knows when lunch is ready and when it is time for Bible Study and hymn singing. Sometimes we sing the old hymns together, and she mouths the words through her tears. "God will take care of you. God will take care of you."

She knows that her roommate is unreasonable and that her helping aide is kind. She knows that she is helpless, and that her family loves her. When she is lucid, she prays. My sister and I pray with her. She prays for strength. She prays not to be unkind. She prays for peacefulness.

A few days ago, after a difficult and frustrating morning that had reduced her to tears and left me steeling myself within, we were sitting on the patio, warming our faces in the weak winter sun. We were sitting face to face, as close as her wheelchair would allow. Her hand in mine, always in mine, gripped hard. She said to me clearly, "You are a blessing to me." I could not hide my tears then.

A friend of mine, who nursed her father through a long illness, told me once that after all is said and done, after the person you are caring for and the person that you thought you were before the caregiving, are both stripped bare, down to the core of humanness, something happens. She said, and I will never forget her words, "All that is left between you is the love."

I continue to see my mother through her journey. We travel together, hands clasped tight against the darkness. She saw me come into the world. I will be with her when she leaves the world. My mother is more peaceful now. And so am I. All that is left between us is the love.

Conclusion

And so, your caregiving journey is finished. You were there for your loved one through months and years of intense suffering and intense intimacy. You were loving. You cared. You were the witness to their final journey. They did not die alone. You were there for them. You have done well.

And now? There is grief and relief and a bittersweet numbness that will give way to a new rebirth for you. Because life never ends. It only changes form.

I was taught this lesson many years ago, when I lived in L.A. and dealt with caregiving, grief, loss, and going forward despite all appearances to the contrary, year after year after year. An Episcopal minister, who was also my spiritual counselor, told me the following when I went to see him about new challenges, those far beyond the death of my son. It seemed to me, at the time we spoke, that the challenges I was facing heralded the loss of all that I had worked for for seven years and the death of all my dreams.

"You are still here," he said, "with all your will and all your spirit. Your true essence can never be taken away from you. Only the form changes. The people you love may leave you. Your possessions, location, creativity, opportunities, all may change. Must change as you develop and grow. As you let go of the past. But you are still here. Everything else may fall away. You are still here."

Only the form changes. In an instant I could see that what looked like the death of all my dreams was simply the dissolving of an old form so that a new form could emerge.

"You CAN walk through this trial by fire," my friend told me. "Your current rage and sorrow are natural responses to these changes in your life. But you will not drown in your emotions. You have come too far for that. Just remember, everything in life changes form. Your loved ones change form, as they go onward into the next stage of their resurrection. Flowers bud and bloom and die and go to earth and are reborn in their next springtime. The cells of your body are born and die and are replaced, miraculously, hour after hour. Everything in life changes form. You are merely entering a new season of your life."

His words echo through me now, after the caregiving. So I'm moving on. I keep moving on. You will too. I promise you. Only the form changes. The love remains.

Welcome to a new season of your life!

APPENDIX A

Legal Forms

Notice of Death-with-Dignity Request
Designation of Health Care Surrogate
Living Will

Following are some sample legal documents needed to assist both the caregiver and the patient in putting affairs in order, and will also assist the patient in expressing her exact wishes. Each state's forms may vary; you should consult with a local attorney about legal issues. The Florida forms are reprinted by permission of Choice in Dying, 200 Varick Street, New York, NY 10014. (212) 366-5540.

Appendix A

Sample
Death with Dignity Direction

TO: My family, my physician, my lawyer, my clergyman;
TO: Any medical facility in whose care I happen to be;
TO: Any individual who may become responsible for my
    health, welfare, or affairs

Death is as much a reality as birth, growth, maturity and old age. It is the one certainty of life. If the time comes when I, _____, can no longer take part in decisions for my own future, let this statement stand as an expression of my wishes, while I am still capable of expressing my wishes.

I, _____, being of sound mind, willfully, and voluntarily make known my desire that my life shall not be artificially prolonged under the circumstances set forth below, and do hereby declare that:

(a) If at any time I should have an incurable injury, disease or illness certified to be a terminal condition by two physicians, and where the application of life-sustaining procedures would serve only to artificially prolong the moment of my death, and where my physician determines that my death is imminent whether or not life-sustaining procedures are utilized, I direct that such procedures be withheld or withdrawn, and that I be permitted to die naturally;

(b) In the absence of my ability to give directions regarding the use of such life-sustaining procedures, it is my intention that this directive shall be honored by my family and physician(s) as the final expression of my legal right to refuse medical or surgical treatment and I accept the consequences from such refusal;

(c) If I have been diagnosed as pregnant, and that diagnosis is known to my physician, this directive shall have no force or effect during the course of my pregnancy;

(d) I understand the full import of this directive and I am emotionally and mentally competent to make this directive.

This directive is made after careful consideration. I hope you who care for me will feel morally bound to follow its mandate. I recognize that this appears to place a heavy responsibility upon you, but it is with the intention of relieving you of such responsibility and of placing it upon myself in accordance with my strong convictions, that this directive is made.

IN WITNESS WHEREOF, I _____ have set my hand this _____ day of _____, 19_____.

_____
(Name)

_____
_____
(Address)

The declarer has been personally known to me and I believe him/her to be of sound mind. I am not related to the declarer, nor will I gain by his/her death. I am not associated with any person or organization who provides health care services to the declarer.

DATED THIS _____ day of _____, 19_____.

_____
WITNESS

_____
WITNESS

(This particular form may not be applicable in your state or circumstances. Please check with a local attorney.)

Appendix A

FLORIDA DESIGNATION OF HEALTH CARE SURROGATE

Name:_____

    (Last)   *(First)*   *(Middle Initial)*

In the event that I have been determined to be incapacitated to provide informed consent for medical treatment and surgical and diagnostic procedures, I wish to designate as my surrogate for health care decisions:

Name:_____
Address:_____
_____ Zip Code:_____
Phone:_____

If my surrogate is unwilling or unable to perform his duties, I wish to designate as my alternate surrogate:

Name:_____
Address:_____
_____ Zip Code:_____
Phone:_____

I fully understand that this designation will permit my designee to make health care decisions and to provide, withhold, or withdraw consent on my behalf; to apply for public benefits to defray the cost of health care; and to authorize my admission to or transfer from a health care facility.

Additional instructions (optional):

I further affirm that this designation is not being made as a condition of treatment or admission to a health care facility. I will notify and send a copy of this document to the following persons other than my surrogate, so they may know who my surrogate is:

PRINT THE NAMES, AND ADDRESSES OF THOSE WHO YOU WANT TO KEEP COPIES OF THIS DOCUMENT

Name: _____
Address: _____

Name: _____
Address: _____

SIGN AND DATE THE DOCUMENT

Signed: _____
Date: _____

WITNESSING PROCEDURE

TWO WITNESSES MUST SIGN AND PRINT THEIR ADDRESSES

Witness 1:
    Signed: _____
    Address: _____

Witness 2:
    Signed: _____
    Address: _____

SAMPLE

Appendix A

FLORIDA LIVING WILL

INSTRUCTIONS

PRINT THE DATE

PRINT YOUR
NAME

Declaration made this ___ day of _____, 19_.

I, _____, willfully and voluntarily make known my desire that my dying not be artificially prolonged under the circumstances set forth below, and I do hereby declare:

If at any time I have a terminal condition and if my attending or treating physician and another consulting physician have determined that there is no medical probability of my recovery from such condition, I direct that life-prolonging procedures be withheld or withdrawn when the application of such procedures would serve only to prolong artificially the process of dying, and that I be permitted to die naturally with only the administration of medication or the performance of any medical procedure deemed necessary to provide me with comfort care or to alleviate pain.

It is my intention that this declaration be honored by my family and physician as the final expression of my legal right to refuse medical or surgical treatment and to accept the consequences for such refusal.

In the event that I have been determined to be unable to provide express and informed consent regarding the withholding, withdrawal, or continuation of life-prolonging procedures, I wish to designate, as my surrogate to carry out the provisions of this declaration:

PRINT THE
NAME, HOME
ADDRESS AND
TELEPHONE
NUMBER OF
YOUR
SURROGATE

Name:_____
Address:_____
_____ Zip Code:_____
Phone:_____

I wish to designate the following person as my alternate surrogate, to carry out the provisions of this declaration should my surrogate be unwilling or unable to act on my behalf:

**PRINT NAME
HOME ADDRESS
AND TELEPHONE
NUMBER OF YOUR
ALTERNATED
SURROGATE**

Name:_____

Address:_____

_____ Zip Code:_____

Phone:_____

**ADD PERSONAL
INSTRUCTIONS
(IF ANY)**

Additional instructions (optional):

I understand the full import of this declaration, and I am emotionally and mentally competent to make this declaration.

**SIGN THE
DOCUMENT**

Signed: _____

**WITNESSING
PROCEDURE**

Witness 1:
        Signed: _____
        Address: _____

**TWO WITNESSES
MUST SIGN AND
PRINT THEIR
ADDRESSES**

Witness 2:
        Signed: _____
        Address: _____

© 1996
CHOICE IN DYING, INC.

Courtesy of **Choice In Dying, Inc.**   6/96
200 Varick Street, New York, NY 10014 212-366-5540

APPENDIX B

Resource Guide

National Organizations Concerned with Health Care and Elder Care

Some of these resources assist current caregivers; they also provide support to older adults in aspects of autonomous living.

American Association of Retired Persons (AARP), 1909 K Street NW, Washington, DC 20049. (202) 872-4700.For a list of brochures write to: Fulfillment, Box 2240, Lakewood, CA 90802. AARP also coordinates "Healthy U.S.," a campaign of political and consumer action and health promotion activities.

Children of Aging Parents, 2761 Trenton Road, Levittown, PA 19056. (215) 945-6900. Offers information on selecting care.

Family Service America, 333 Seventh Avenue, New York, NY 10001. (212) 967-2740. Will provide information on social service agencies in your area.

National Association of Area Agencies on Aging, 600 Maryland Avenue SW, Washington, DC 20024. (202) 484-7520. Will provide you with the address of your local area agency on aging.

National Council on the Aging, 600 Maryland Avenue SW, West Wing 100, Washington, DC 20024. (202) 479-1200. Provides information and resources on caregiving and long-term care. Write for a list of their publications. You can contact the National Institute on Adult Day Care at the same address.

National Federation of Interfaith Volunteer Caregivers, 105 Mary's Avenue, Kingston, NY 12041. (914) 331-2198. Provides transportation, minimal in-home help, and visiting services to elderly as well as referrals to other relevant community services.

National Shared Housing Resource Center (NSHRC), 6344 Greene Street, Philadelphia, PA 19144. (215) 848-1220. Information and referrals.

Older Women's League (OWL), 730 Eleventh Street NW, Suite 300, Washington, DC 20001. (202) 783-6686. A national grass-roots advocacy organization concerned with issues of importance to midlife and older women.

Senior Service Corporation, 354 Nod Hill Road, Wilton, CT 06897. (203) 834-1644. Public corporation that provides products and services for elders.

The following agencies vary state by state with regard to laws and practices. Please check the yellow pages in your area phone book for up-to-date listings for your area.

Listings of VNA (Visiting Nurses Association) resources are also available state by state. Some areas list the VNA resources under "Home Health Care Agencies," or a similar heading. And some VNA resources are affiliated with local hospitals.

Supportive Services for Older Adults
Independence Plus Agencies
Senior Partners

Senior Support Services
Prime Time Seniors
Service Consortium for Older Persons
United Senior Care

Self-Help Clearinghouses

These clearinghouses can help you find a free support group in your area before, during, and after the caregiving.

National Self-Help Clearinghouse	(201) 625-7101
Self-Help Center	(312) 328-0470
National Clearinghouse	(212) 642-2944

Directory of State Insurance Departments and Agencies on Aging

Each state has its own laws and regulations governing all types of insurance. The insurance offices, listed in the left column, are responsible for enforcing those laws, as well as providing the public with information about insurance. The agencies on aging, listed in the right column, are responsible for coordinating services for older persons. The middle column of the directory lists the telephone number to call for insurance counseling services. Calls to an 800 number listed in this directory are free when made within the respective state.

INSURANCE DEPARTMENT	INSURANCE COUNSELING	AGENCIES ON AGING

ALABAMA

Insurance Dept.	1-800-243-5463	Commission on Aging
Consumer Service Div.		770 Washington Ave.,
135 South Union St.		Suite 470
P.O. Box 303351		P.O. Box 301851
Montgomery, AL 36130-3351		Montgomery, AL 36130
(334) 269-3550		1-800-243-5463
		(334) 242-5743

ALASKA

Division of Insurance	1-800-478-6065	Older Alaskans Comm.
800 E. Dimond, Suite 560	(907) 562-7249	P.O. Box 110209
Anchorage, AK 99515		Juneau, AK 99811-0209
(907) 349-1230		(907) 465-3250

AMERICAN SAMOA

Insurance Department		Territorial Admin. on Aging
Office of the Governor		Government of American Samoa
Pago Pago, AS 96799		Pago Pago, AS 96799
011 (684) 633-4116		011 (684) 633-1252

INSURANCE DEPARTMENT	INSURANCE COUNSELING	AGENCIES ON AGING
ARIZONA		
Insurance Department Consumer Affairs Div. 2910 N. 44th Street Phoenix, AZ 85018 (602) 912-8444	1-800-432-4040 (602) 542-6595	Dept. of Economic Security Aging and Adult Admin. 1789 W. Jefferson St. Phoenix, AZ 85007 (602) 542-4446
ARKANSAS		
Insurance Department Seniors Insurance Network 1123 S. University Ave., Suite 400 Little Rock, AR 72204 1-800-852-5494	1-800-852-5494 (501) 686-2940	Division of Aging and Adult Services 1417 Donaghey Plaza South P.O. Box 1437/Slot 1412 Little Rock, AR 72203-1437
CALIFORNIA		
Insurance Department Consumer Services Div. 300 S. Spring Street Los Angeles, CA 90013 (213) 897-8921	1-800-927-4357 (916) 323-7315	Department of Aging 1600 K Street Sacramento, CA 95814 (916) 322-3887

Insurance Department	Insurance Counseling	Agencies on Aging

COLORADO

Insurance Division	1-800-544-9181	Aging and Adult
1560 Broadway,	(303) 894-7499	Services
Suite 850	ext. 356	Dept. of Social
Denver, CO 80202		Services
(303) 894-7499, ext. 356		1575 Sherman St.,
		4th Floor
		Denver, CO 80203-
		1714

COMMONWEALTH OF THE NORTHERN MARIANA ISLANDS

Department of
    Community
    and Cultural Affairs
Civic Center
Commonwealth of
    the Northern
    Mariana Islands
Saipan, CM 96950
(607) 234-6011

CONNECTICUT

Insurance Department	1-800-443-9946	Elderly Services Div.
P.O. Box 816		175 Main Street
Hartford, CT 06143-0816		Hartford, CT 06106
(203) 297-3800		1-800-443-9946

INSURANCE DEPARTMENT	INSURANCE COUNSELING	AGENCIES ON AGING

DELAWARE

Insurance Department
Rodney Building
841 Silver Lake Blvd.
Dover, DE 19904
1-800-281-8611
(302) 739-4251
	1-800-336-9500	Division of Aging
		Dept. of Health and
		  Social Services
		1901 N. DuPont
		  Highway
		Annex Admin. Bldg.,
		  2nd Floor
		New Castle, DE
		  19720
		(302) 577-4791

DISTRICT OF COLUMBIA

Insurance Department
Consumer and Professional
  Services Bureau
441 4th Street, NW,
  Suite 850 North
Washington, DC 20001
	(202) 994-7463	Office of Aging
		441 4th Street, NW,
		  9th Floor
		Washington, DC
		  20001
		(202) 724-5626
		(202) 724-5622

FEDERATED STATES OF MICRONESIA

		State Agency on Aging
		Office of Health
		  Services
		Federated States of
		  Micronesia
		Ponape, E.C.I. 96941

INSURANCE DEPARTMENT	INSURANCE COUNSELING	AGENCIES ON AGING

FLORIDA

Dept. of Insurance
200 E. Gaines Street
Tallahassee, FL 32399-0300
(904) 922-3100

(904) 922-2073

Department of Elder
  Affairs
1317 Winewood Blvd.,
Building 1, Room 317
Tallahassee, FL
  32399-0700
(904) 922-5297

GEORGIA

Insurance Dept.
2 Martin L. King, Jr., Dr.
716 West Tower
Atlanta, GA 30334
(404) 656-2056

1-800-669-8387

Division of Aging
  Services
Dept. of Human
  Resources
2 Peachtree St., NW,
  Room 18.403
Atlanta, GA 30303
(404) 657-5258

GUAM

Insurance Dept.
Dept. of Revenue
  and Taxation
378 Chalan San Antonio
Tamunning, Guam 96911
011 (671) 477-5144

Division of Senior
  Citizens
Dept. of Public
  Health and Social
  Services
P.O. Box 2816
Agana, Guam 96910
011 (671) 632-4141

INSURANCE DEPARTMENT	INSURANCE COUNSELING	AGENCIES ON AGING

HAWAII

Dept. of Commerce and Consumer Affairs
Insurance Division
P.O. Box 3614
Honolulu, HI 96811
(808) 586-2790

(808) 586-0100

Executive Office on Aging
335 Merchant Street, Room 241
Honolulu, HI 96813
(808) 586-0100

IDAHO

Insurance Dept.
SHIBA Program
700 W. State St., 3rd Floor
Boise, ID 83720-0043

S.W.: 1-800-247-4422
N.: 1-800-488-5725
S.E.: 1-800-488-5764
C.: 1-800-488-5731

Office on Aging
Statehouse, Rm. 108
Boise, ID 83720
(208) 334-3833

ILLINOIS

Insurance Dept.
320 W. Washington St., 4th Floor
Springfield, IL 62767
(217) 7820-4515

1-800-548-9034

Dept. of Aging
421 E. Capitol Ave.
Springfield, IL 62701
(217) 785-3356

INDIANA

Insurance Dept.
311 W. Washington St., Suite 300
Indianapolis, IN 46204
1-800-622-4461
(317) 232-2395

1-800-452-4800

Div. of Aging and Home Services
402 W. Washington St.
P.O. Box 7083
Indianapolis, IN 46207-7083
1-800-545-7763
(317) 281-5187

INSURANCE DEPARTMENT	INSURANCE COUNSELING	AGENCIES ON AGING

IOWA

Insurance Division
Lucas State Office Bldg.
E. 12th and Grand Sts.,
  6th Floor
Des Moines, IA 50319
(515) 281-5705

1-800-281-5705

Dept. of Elder Affairs
Jewett Bldg., Ste. 236
914 Grand Avenue
Des Moines, IA 50309
(515) 281-5187

KANSAS

Insurance Dept.
420 S.W. 9th Street
Topeka, KS 66612
1-800-432-2484
(913) 296-3071

1-800-432-3535

Dept. on Aging
150 S. Docking State
  Office Building
915 S.W. Harrison
Topeka, KS 66612-
  1500
(913) 296-4986

KENTUCKY

Insurance Dept.
215 W. Main Street
P.O. Box 517
Frankfort, KY 40602
(502) 564-3630

1-800-372-2973

Div. of Aging Services
Cabinet for Human
  Resources
275 E. Main St.,
  5th Floor West
Frankfort, KY 40601
(502) 564-6930

INSURANCE DEPARTMENT	INSURANCE COUNSELING	AGENCIES ON AGING

LOUISIANA

Senior Health Insurance Information Program (SHIIP) Insurance Department P.O. Box 94214 Baton Rouge, LA 70804-9214 (504) 342-5301

1-800-259-5301

Governor's Office of Elderly Affairs 4550 North Blvd. P.O. Box 80374 Baton Rouge, LA 70896-0374 (504) 925-1700

MAINE

Bureau of Insurance Consumer Division State House, Station 34 Augusta, ME 04333 (207) 582-8707

1-800-750-5353

Bureau of Elder and Adult Services State House, Station 11 Augusta, ME 04333 (207) 624-5335

MARYLAND

Insurance Admin. Complaints and Investigation Unit—Life and Health 501 St. Paul Place Baltimore, MD 21202-2272 (410) 333-2793 (410) 333-2770

1-800-243-3425

Office on Aging 301 W. Preston St., Room 1004 Baltimore, MD 21201 (410) 225-1102

INSURANCE DEPARTMENT	INSURANCE COUNSELING	AGENCIES ON AGING

MASSACHUSETTS

Insurance Division Consumer Services Section 470 Atlantic Ave. Boston, MA 02210-2223 (617) 521-7777	1-800-882-2003 (617) 727-7750	Executive Office of Elder Affairs 1 Ashburton Place, 5th Floor Boston, MA 02108 1-800-882-2003 (617) 727-7750

MICHIGAN

Insurance Bureau P.O. Box 30220 Lansing, MI 48909 (517) 373-0240 *(general assistance)* (517) 335-1702 *(senior issues)*	(517) 373-8230	Office of Services to the Aging 611 W. Ottawa Street P.O. Box 30026 Lansing, MI 48909 (517) 373-8230

MINNESOTA

Insurance Department Dept. of Commerce 133 E. 7th Street St. Paul, MN 55101-2362 (612) 296-4026	1-800-882-6262	Board on Aging Human Services Bldg. 4th Floor 444 Lafayette Road St. Paul, MN 55155-3843 (612) 296-2770

INSURANCE DEPARTMENT	INSURANCE COUNSELING	AGENCIES ON AGING
MISSISSIPPI		
Insurance Dept. Consumer Assistance Division P.O. Box 79 Jackson, MS 39205 (601) 359-3569	1-800-948-3090	Div. of Aging and Adult Services 750 N. State Street Jackson, MS 39202 1-800-948-3090
MISSOURI		
Dept. of Insurance Consumer Services Section P.O. Box 690 Jefferson City, MO 65102-0690 1-800-726-7390 (314) 751-2640	1-800-390-3330	Division of Aging Dept. of Social Services P.O. Box 1337 615 Howerton Court Jefferson City, MO 65102-1337 (314) 751-3082
MONTANA		
Insurance Dept. 126 N. Sanders Mitchell Bldg., Room 270 P.O. Box 4009 Helena, MT 59601 (406) 444-2040	1-800-332-2272	Office on Aging 48 N. Last Chance Gulch P.O. Box 8005 Helena, MT 59620 1-800-332-2272 (406) 444-5900

Insurance Department	Insurance Counseling	Agencies on Aging

NEBRASKA

Insurance Dept.
Terminal Building
941 "O" St., Suite 400
Lincoln, NE 68508
(402) 471-2201

(402) 471-4506

Dept. on Aging
State Office Building
301 Centennial Mall
   South
Lincoln, NE 68509-
   5044
(402) 471-2306

NEVADA

Dept. of Business
   and Industry
Div. of Insurance
1665 Hot Springs Rd.,
   Suite 152
Carson City, NV 89710
(702) 687-4270
1-800-992-0900

1-800-307-4444
(702) 367-1218

Dept. of Human
   Resources
Div. for Aging Services
340 N. 11th St.,
   Suite 114
Las Vegas, NV 89101
(702) 486-3545

NEW HAMPSHIRE

Insurance Dept.
Life and Health Div.
169 Manchester St.
Concord, NH 03301
1-800-852-3416
(603) 271-2261

1-800-852-3388
(603) 271-4642

Dept. of Health and
   Human Services
Div. of Elderly and
   Adult Services
State Office Park S.
115 Pleasant Street
Annex Building No. 1
Concord, NH 03301
(603) 271-4680

INSURANCE DEPARTMENT	INSURANCE COUNSELING	AGENCIES ON AGING

NEW JERSEY

Insurance Dept. 20 West State Street Roebling Building, CN 325 Trenton, NJ 08625 (609) 292-5363	1-800-792-8820	Dept. Of Community Affairs Division on Aging 101 S. Broad Street, CN 807 Trenton, NJ 08625- 0807 1-800-792-8820 (609) 984-3951

NEW MEXICO

Insurance Dept. P.O. Drawer 1269 Santa Fe, NM 87504-1269 (505) 827-4500	1-800-432-2080	State Agency on Aging La Villa Rivera Bldg. 224 E. Palace Ave. Santa Fe, NM 87501 1-800-432-2080 (505) 827-7640

NEW YORK

Insurance Dept. 160 West Broadway New York, NY 10013 (212) 602-0203 *Outside of New York City:* 1-800-342-3736	1-800-333-4114 *NYC area:* (212) 869-3850	State Office for the Aging 2 Empire State Plaza Albany, NY 12223- 0001 1-800-342-9871 (518) 474-5731

INSURANCE DEPARTMENT	INSURANCE COUNSELING	AGENCIES ON AGING

NORTH CAROLINA

Insurance Dept.   1-800-443-9354
Seniors' Health Insurance
  Information Program
  (SHIIP)
P.O. Box 26387
Raleigh, NC 27611
(919) 733-0111 *(SHIIP)*
1-800-662-7777
(consumer services)

Division of Aging
693 Palmer Drive
Caller Box 29531
Raleigh, NC 27626-
  0531
(919) 733-3983

NORTH DAKOTA

Insurance Dept.   1-800-247-0560
Senior Health
  Insurance Counseling
600 E. Boulevard
Bismarck, ND 58505-
  0320
1-800-247-0560
(701) 328-2440

Dept. of Human
  Services Aging
  Services Div.
P.O. Box 7070
Bismarck, ND
  58507-7070
1-800-755-8521
(701) 328-2577

OHIO

Insurance Dept.   1-800-686-1578
Consumer Services Div.
2100 Stella Court
Columbus, OH
  43215-1067
1-800-686-1526
(614) 644-2673

Department of Aging
50 W. Broad Street,
  9th Floor
Columbus, OH
  43215-5928
1-800-282-1206
(614) 466-1221

INSURANCE DEPARTMENT	INSURANCE COUNSELING	AGENCIES ON AGING

OKLAHOMA

	(405) 521-6628	

Insurance Dept.
P.O. Box 53408
Oklahoma City, OK
  73152-3408
(405) 521-6628
		Dept. of Human
		  Services
		Aging Services Div.
		312 N.E. 28th Street
		Oklahoma City, OK
		  73125
		(405) 521-2327

OREGON

Dept. of Consumer	1-800-722-4134	Dept. of Human

and Business Services
Senior Health Insurance
Benefits Assistance
470 Labor and
  Industries Bldg.
Salem, OR 97310
(503) 378-4484
		Resources
		Senior and Disabled
		  Services Division
		500 Summer St., NE,
		  2nd Floor
		Salem, OR 97310-
		  1015
		1-800-232-3020
		(503) 945-5811

PALAU

		State Agency on Aging
		Dept. of Social Services Republic of Palau Koror, Palau 96940

INSURANCE DEPARTMENT	INSURANCE COUNSELING	AGENCIES ON AGING

PENNSYLVANIA

	1-800-783-7067	
Insurance Dept. Consumer Services Bureau 1321 Strawberry Sq. Harrisburg, PA 17120 (717) 787-2317		Department of Aging "Apprise" Health Insurance Counseling and Assistance 400 Market Street State Office Building Harrisburg, PA 17101 1-800-783-7067

PUERTO RICO

	(809) 721-5710	
Office of the Commissioner of Insurance P.O. Box 8330 San Juan, PR 00910-8330 (809) 722-8686		Governor's Office of Elderly Affairs Gericulture Commission Box 11398 Santurce, PR 00910 (809) 722-2429

REPUBLIC OF THE MARSHALL ISLANDS

State Agency on Aging
Dept. of Social
Services
Republic of the
Marshall Islands
Marjuro, Marshall
Islands 96960

INSURANCE DEPARTMENT	INSURANCE COUNSELING	AGENCIES ON AGING

RHODE ISLAND

Insurance Division 233 Richmond St., Suite 233 Providence, RI 02903-4233 (401) 277-2223	1-800-322-2880	Dept. of Elderly Affairs 160 Pine Street Providence, RI 02903 (401) 277-2858

SOUTH CAROLINA

Dept. of Insurance Consumer Services Sec. P.O. Box 100105 Columbia, SC 29202-3105 (803) 737-6180	1-800-868-9095	Division on Aging 202 Arbor Lake Dr., Suite 301 Columbia, SC 29223-4554 (803) 737-7500

SOUTH DAKOTA

Insurance Dept. 500 E. Capitol Ave. Pierre, SD 57501-5070 (605) 773-3563	(605) 773-3656	Office of Adult Services and Aging 700 Governors Drive Pierre, SD 57501-2291 (605) 773-3656

INSURANCE DEPARTMENT	INSURANCE COUNSELING	AGENCIES ON AGING

TENNESSEE

| Dept. of Commerce and Insurance Insurance Assistance Office 500 James Robertson Pkwy, 4th Floor Nashville, TN 37243 1-800-525-2816 (615) 741-4955 | 1-800-525-2816 | Commission on Aging Andrew Jackson Bldg. 500 Deaderick St., 9th Floor Nashville, TN 37243 (615) 741-2056 |

TEXAS

| Dept. of Insurance Complaints Resolution, MC 111-1A 333 Guadalupe Street P.O. Box 149091 Austin, TX 78714-9091 1-800-252-3439 (512) 463-6500 | 1-800-252-3439 | Dept. on Aging P.O. Box 12786 (78711) 1949 IH 35 South Austin, TX 76741 1-800-252-9240 (512) 444-2727 |

UTAH

| Insurance Dept. Consumer Services 3110 State Office Bldg. Salt Lake City, UT 84114-6901 1-800-429-3805 | 1-800-606-0608 | Div. of Aging and Adult Services 120 North 200 West Salt Lake City, UT 84103 1-800-606-0608 |

INSURANCE DEPARTMENT	INSURANCE COUNSELING	AGENCIES ON AGING

VERMONT

Dept. of Banking and Insurance Consumer Complaint Div. 89 Main St., Drawer 20 Montpelier, VT 05620-3101 (802) 828-3302	1-800-828-3302	Dept. of Aging and Disabilities Waterbury Complex 103 S. Main Street Waterbury, VT 05671-2301 (802) 241-2400

VIRGINIA

Bureau of Insurance Consumer Services Div. 1300 E. Main Street P.O. Box 1157 Richmond, VA 23209 1-800-552-7945 (804) 371-9741	1-800-663-5565	Dept. for the Aging 700 Centre, 10th Fl. 700 E. Franklin St. Richmond, VA 23219-2327 1-800-552-4464 (804) 225-2271

VIRGIN ISLANDS

Insurance Dept. Kongens Gade No. 18 St. Thomas, VI 00802 (809) 774-2991	(809) 774-2991	Senior Citizen Affairs Div. Dept. of Human Services 19 Estate Diamond Fredericksted St. Croix, VI 00840 (809) 662-0939

INSURANCE DEPARTMENT	INSURANCE COUNSELING	AGENCIES ON AGING

WASHINGTON

Insurance Dept.	1-800-397-4422	Aging and Adult

Insurance Dept.
4224 6th Ave. SE.,
    Bldg. 4
P.O. Box 40256
Lacey, WA 98504-0256
1-800-562-6900
(360) 753-7300

1-800-397-4422

Aging and Adult
    Services Admin.
Dept. of Social and
    Health Services
P.O. Box 45050
Olympia, WA 98504-
    5050
(360) 586-3768

WEST VIRGINIA

Insurance Dept.
Consumer Service Div.
2019 Washington St., East
P.O. Box 50540
Charleston, WV 25305-0540
1-800-642-9004
1-800-435-7381 *(hearing impaired)*
(304) 558-3386

1-800-558-3317

Commission on Aging
State Capitol Complex
Holly Grove
1900 Kanawha Blvd.,
    East
Charleston, WV
    25305-0160
(304) 558-3317

WISCONSIN

Insurance Dept.
Complaints Dept.
P.O. Box 7873
Madison, WI 53707
1-800-236-8517
(608) 266-0103

1-800-242-1060

Board on Aging and
    Long-term Care
214 N. Hamilton St.
Madison, WI 53703
1-800-242-1060
(608) 266-8944

INSURANCE DEPARTMENT	INSURANCE COUNSELING	AGENCIES ON AGING

WYOMING

Insurance Dept.	1-800-438-5768	Division on Aging
Herschler Building		Hathaway Building
122 W. 25th Street		2300 Capitol Ave.,
Cheyenne, WY 82002		Room 139
1-800-438-5768		Cheyenne, WY 82002
(307) 777-7401		1-800-442-2766
		(307) 777-7986

Acknowledgments and Permissions

Grateful acknowledgment is made to the following for permission to reprint the following material:

Excerpted material "Please Listen" by Dr. Ray Houghton from *Stepping Stones to Grief Recovery* by Deborah Roth. IBS Press, Santa Monica, California. Copyright © 1988 by Deborah Roth. Reprinted by permission of the author.

Thanks to Chelsea Psychotherapy Associates, NYC, for permission to reprint excerpts from "When a Friend Has AIDS" and "Saying Good-bye to Someone You Love." Authors: Dixie Beckham, Diego Lopez, Luis Palacios-Jimenez, Vincent Patti and Michael Shernoff.

"Forgiveness and Caring," including: "Folding the Sheets," "Forgiving the System," and "Preventive Forgiveness," by Betty-Clare Moffatt originally appeared in *Journey Toward Forgiveness: Finding Your Way Home*. MasterMedia, Ltd., New York, 1995. Reprinted by permission of MasterMedia, Ltd.

Excerpt from "Gentle Ghosts" from *Opening to Miracles* by Betty-Clare Moffatt reprinted with the permission of Wildcat Canyon Press. Copyright © 1995 by BettyClare Moffatt.

Excerpted material "All of the Laughter, All of the Tears" and "Symptoms of Loss" from *Stepping Stones to Grief Recovery* by Deborah Roth. IBS Press, Santa Monica, California. Copyright © 1988 by Deborah Roth. Reprinted by permission of the author.

Excerpt from "Family Possessions" from *A Soulworker's Companion* by BettyClare Moffatt reprinted by permission of Wildcat Canyon Press. Copyright © 1996 by BettyClare Moffatt.

"Saying Good-bye to Someone You Love" by Chelsea Psychotherapy Associates originally appeared in *Gifts for the Living* by BettyClare Moffatt. IBS Press, Santa Monica, California. Copyright © 1988 by BettyClare Moffatt.

"The Dying Person's Bill of Rights" by E. M. Baulch excerpted from *Extended Health Care at Home*. Copyright © 1988 by Evelyn Baulch. Reprinted by permission of Celestial Arts, P.O. Box 7123, Berkeley.

Excerpt from *When Someone You Love Has AIDS* by BettyClare Moffatt. Originally published by NAL.

Poetry excerpts of pages 132 and 142 are from "Do Not Go Gentle into That Night" by Dylan Thomas, 1952.

Portions of "I Want to Go Home" by Mary Schramski appeared in a slightly different form in *Personal Transformation* magazine, Winter 1994. Used by permission of *Personal Transformation*.

Poem on page 174 is from an unknown author. It is reprinted from *Being Human in the Face of Death* by Deborah Roth. IBS Press, Santa Monica, California. Reprinted by permission of the author. Copyright © 1989 by Deborah Roth.

"Throwing Stones" from *Soulwork* by BettyClare Moffatt reprinted with permission of Wildcat Canyon Press. Copyright © 1994 by BettyClare Moffatt.

Thanks to National Association of Insurance Commissioners and the U.S. Department of Health and Human Services for Medicare and Long-Term Care Insurance Information.

Thanks to Choice in Dying, 200 Varick Street, New York, New York 10014 for permission to reprint the Florida Advance Directives.

Contributors

Chelsea Psychotherapy Associates
Helen Thomas Cook
Connie Courtney
Diane Harvey
David Kessler
Margie Ann Nicola
Carol W. Parrish-Harra
Rita Robinson
Deborah Roth
Mary Schramski
Joey Shea
William L. Welsch—appendix material
Laurie Williams